This Book is fo

This book is for you if you are suffering, physically or emotionally. If you're not being heard, if you think you are invisible, if you get nervous in social situations, overwhelmed and at times feel sad and alone. You are certainly NOT alone, you are simply human like everyone else. Don't panic though, for this is where the magic is....

Learning how to be released from suffering - physically and energetically requires you to discover your internal truth and express this to your world. This is the beginnings of a beautiful and life fulfilling ripple effect. Expressing your world, to the world, with power and honesty.

This book is dedicated to the silent, suffering superheroes out there. Those who have a burning desire to have a voice and be acknowledged, not just by those who are close, but by the wider community. You have something to contribute, so much so that it makes your heart flutter, your belly burn, and your cheeks go red when you are faced with an opportunity to express yourself.

What people are saying...

Carly is an expert in her field. Not only can she help find & treat the problem through her knowledge and techniques, but she gives an explanation to the root cause of the problem. I highly recommend her.

Lisa Festa
Mum & business owner

The online I AM WELLness plan gives me the chance to rejuvenate my energy and alleviate physical tension. With just 10 minutes of guided self-care a day, I feel like I have been to the spa. Carly has helped me learn the importance and effectiveness of 'me time.'

Natalie Mansford, Specialist Physiotherapist

Carly's online I AM WELLness plan is refreshing and has been an invaluable tool for coping with the mental demands of family and workload. Just a few minutes per day is required to allow me to focus on myself and my wellbeing. Recipes, self-massage techniques, yogic breath, and meditations allowed me to holistically immerse in some much-needed me-time, which benefitted all those around me too.

Ciara Hynes, business owner

Absolutely incredible holistic health training. I would highly recommend Carly and her services.

Dr Jasmina Paul, Clinic Director at Aesthetics Glow

What people are saying...

Amazing training. Thank you, Carly, for your knowledge and inspiration. Great to be taught by a true professional.

Justine Bunting, holistic business owner

'I have had the great pleasure of knowing Carly for 10 years, and it has been amazing to see her transform from a very skilled, connected spa therapist, to become the revered multi-faceted wellness guru she is today. Carly has a beautiful soul and has a fantastic wealth of knowledge, teaching her clients and training teams across the globe with integrity,love and compassion.

Julie Brown, working mum & owner of Boutique Wellbeing

The yoga classes and retreat I have taken with Carly opened my eyes to a spiritual connection I had never been able to fully tap in to. The yoga I practice today has grown from the seeds she planted. It's wonderful to finally be able to connect my body and mind. Being able to unravel who you are is very exciting. Thank you Carly.

Victoria Young, working mum of two

I first started working with Carly around 3 years ago. I have learned so much about myself through Carly's teachings about so much more than yoga. Carly's showed me how to balance my body, to notice when things are a little "out of whack" and taught me the importance of slowing down, taking time and how to find balance in my body again. You won't regret working with Carly.

What people are saying...

She works in a truly holistic manner. She not only listens but hears you. She will see you as the individual that you are.

Helen Discombe, working mum, birth and post-natal doula

Carly is incredibly caring and compassionate, a natural healer whose experience and willingness to help people really shines through.

I have learnt so much through my practice with her. Her Ayurvedic knowledge and yoga teachings, along with life affirming mantras, have been an intrinsic part of my spiritual growth.

Amanda Farmer, Priestess of Gaia

I have been to numerous therapists, doctors, and physios and none of them have worked! After one treatment with Carly I feel better already, and the pain has significantly reduced!! Thank you so much!

Suzanna Coffey, Senior corporate VIP travel consultant

Carly is a true gem - a spirited teacher and compassionate therapist, insightful and supportive, sensitive and fun. Carly has a beautiful way of making everyone feel special.

Luisa Anderson
Director of Spa, Four Seasons Hotels & Resorts

About the author

I AM unwilling to I AM willing
I AM unworthy to I AM worthy
I AM unwell to I AM WELLness

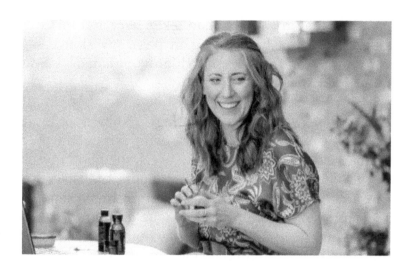

Carly has 15 years' experience in holistic health, integrated therapy and training. Founder of the I AM WELLness community, online self-care course and women's wellness clinic. Carly consults and educates for learning and development companies and wellness brands and studies human psychology at The University of Oxford.

"My journey to wellness has been bumpy and disheartening. Especially when I realised that no-one but me can take responsibility for my health and happiness.

"For a long time, anxiety ruled my life. Add in a debilitating knee injury, a major road traffic accident, a thyroid condition, and one might say my nervous system was shot to pieces! In this period of my life, I didn't know how to separate my best intentions from the thoughts and feelings that were influencing me.

"To comfort my confused self, I would overindulge. To vent my frustration, I would have regular emotional outbursts only fueling my existing hormone imbalances. I realised that my anxiety had taken over and this was the cause of my body being in pain, my skin being unbalanced and my mood highly agitated. I was suffering with chronic stress.

"So, I went to my default settings - known as fight, flight, freeze. I switched off from being present! I would feel like everything was OK one week then find myself working 14-hour days in the wellness industry that aims to promote work-life balance. It made no sense to me. Throw in becoming a new wife and a new mum and enough was enough. I felt anxious, confused and completely sick and tired. In fact, one of my classic lines to this day is 'I feel sick'!

"That's right, even when you have been living and breathing wellness work, being your best self and helping others do the same, you still have off days! My private and professional world of self-discovery was ultimately triggered by a painful past full of self-doubt. In a nutshell, I realised that we simply are what we do consistently. Therefore, health and happiness are not something you magically get and keep forever, rather the gateway to real transformation is in simple daily rituals."

Join the member's area - access your free audio meditation or enrol on the I AM WELLness 25-day plan here - carlychamberlain.podia.com

Join the community - @carlyiamwellness

Work with me - iamwellnesssolution@gmail.com / linkedin.com/in/carly-chamberlain / Facebook - @carlychamberlainwellness

Dedication

To you.

May you find one small wellness ritual to practice

every day. The one that weaves you together through

all the traumas and shifts in your life.

May you honour your body and nurture your soul

from a place of worthiness and love.

May you become a beautiful tapestry of truth.

Acknowledgements

To my husband - the man who says few words and gives unconditionally.

To my children – who remind me every day to laugh and be present.

To my parents - there are no words. You are my life and my light.

To my brothers - who I will look up to forever.

To my friends - for all the fun and all the listening.

To my clients, students, readers and colleagues - who have supported and inspired me on this journey.

To Jeremy Kavanagh - for being the best coach who always holds me accountable to my word.

To Melissa Kay - for helping me see this book through the reader's eyes and for sharing your writing talent with me.

To Chris Day and the team at Filament Publishing - for your expertise and patience.

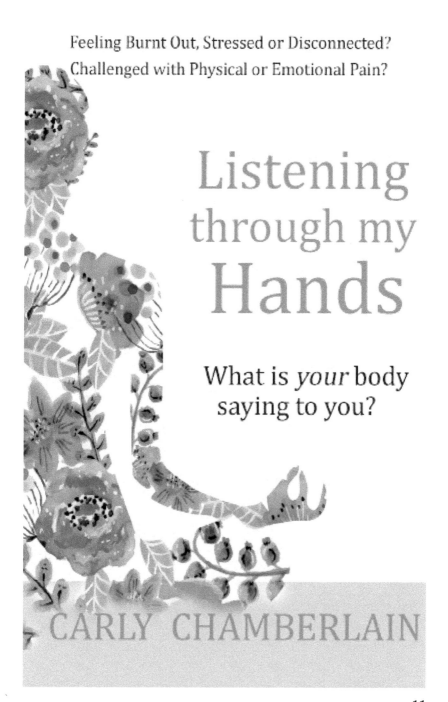

Feeling Burnt Out, Stressed or Disconnected?
Challenged with Physical or Emotional Pain?

Listening
through my
Hands

What is *your* body
saying to you?

CARLY CHAMBERLAIN

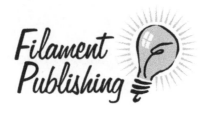

Published by

Filament Publishing Ltd
16, Croydon Road, Beddington,
Croydon, Surrey CR0 4PA
www.filamentublishing.com
email: info@filamentpublishing.com
+44(0)20 8688 2598

"Listening through my Hands"
by Carly Chamberlain
ISBN   978-1-913623-16-6

Printed in the UK by 4Edge

Cover Photo: Katherine Yiannaki

Table of Contents

My discovery   15

What is this book for   17

How to use this book   19

I AM great – believe it or not   20

I AM mother   26

'I AM too little of this and too much of that…   31

Trauma memory 1 - I AM hateful   37

Trauma memory 2 - I AM powerless   41

Trauma memory 3 - I AM unloved   45

Trauma memory 4 - I AM torn   49

I AM born   55

I AM letting go   63

I AM WELLness   70

I AM accepted   77

I AM my head   80

YOU ARE matter and mind   85

YOU ARE joy spark   92

YOU ARE energy   102

YOU ARE a gift to yourself   111

Element - Earth   112

Element - Water   117

Element - Fire   121

Element - Air   124

Element - Space   127

YOU ARE a ritual   130

Step 1 - Affirm   132

Step 2 - Self Massage   140

Step 3 – Movement and breath   148

Step 4 – Fuel   161

Step 5 – Self care   165

YOU ARE unravelling   171

YOU ARE a universe   177

'YOU ARE '   182

References   185

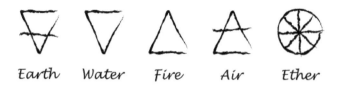

Earth   Water   Fire   Air   Ether

My Discovery...

When we are faced with life's circumstances that appear to be beyond our control, we are engulfed by our primitive survival mode. This mode is fear-based; our comfort zone that does not allow any access to believing we have a choice in the matter. We become even more controlling and more scared; grabbing onto the smallest strings of familiarity that we can find. Even if our circumstances are utterly awful and quite obviously 'beyond our control', we still have a vital part to play in how the situation we face presents itself to us, our world and our future lifestyle habits. Everything is just a matter of perspective.

Where there is control, there is comfort! How bold would it be if we dared to be totally out of control and totally uncomfortable? Scary thought yes? When I say this, I don't mean going on a three-day binge or ranting and raving as you please. Don't mistake control with being irresponsible or giving in to your desires. Control and discipline are two very different things.

I am talking about looking at the situation with an approach we haven't learned yet. To do this we first need to be WILLING. Secondly, we need to commit to putting aside any opinion, judgment, fact, or conclusion we already have about the situation and potential approach. We must commit to be a blank canvas and to restrain ourselves from piping up when we think we have all the answers (or believe there are no answers). We must learn to 'BE' in the situation. Feeling what we are feeling, hearing what we are hearing, seeing what we are seeing, tasting what we are tasting, smelling what we are smelling. Tuning into the five simple human sensory responses and just being with it. This is the gateway to something profound. The five senses correlate to the five Universal Elements.

Earth = smell.
Water = taste.
Fire = sight.
Air = touch.
Space = hearing.

These elements are what make up our human form and what makes up the universe- no coincidence there!

When we practice the simplicity of 'being' with our senses, we learn that in any given situation or terrible circumstance in our life, we can become the witness of it; the observer of the senses, watching them respond as they so instinctively do.

With more practice, we will start to become acutely aware that our identity, our personality and our physical form lives in a space that 'we' the being, the living energy, the life force are no longer attached to. Confidently unattached as opposed to detached and numb. We are no longer governed by our survival mode, yet we are still safe and free. Finding this space is the beginning of our evolution.

What is this book for?

Through the practice of multi-disciplinary body therapy, energy work, yogic and ayurvedic philosophy, I have trained and treated close to 2000 people with chronic and acute physical pain, and emotional or mental health concerns. My work ranges from offering luxurious three-hour body rituals and therapy sessions to the super-rich, to spending three weeks in deep immersion training with the most underprivileged therapists, who work 12-hour shifts in a five-star spa, thousands of miles from home. The main things I have learned from being a hands-on practitioner and trainer is that whatever is happening physically is intimately connected to the mind and energy field - our life force. No matter your money, power or status.

Learning to palpate another person's physical body to facilitate energetic recovery and healing is truly remarkable. Over time, and several hundreds of hours of touch therapy, my sensory neurons and subtle intuition have become attuned to other people's aliveness or lack of aliveness. I have become a witness to the powerful recognition that the mind/body relationship is in full connection with our individual and collective energy; this is the catalyst for achieving balance and fulfillment in life and most importantly, for our true self to be freed up, celebrated and heard.

During this process I have also become witness to the consequences (as a result of biochemical changes) that take place when the mind/body are disconnected. Through my own physical injuries and emotional traumas, I have learned to apply everyday rituals to my life in order to repeatedly return home to harmony.

17

This book is my communication, in words, of the many experiences I have had through my hands, in the treatment room, in training others and in my own encounters - to practice a truly holistic lifestyle. Getting to know the 'I' underneath I and for you to get to know the 'you' underneath you.

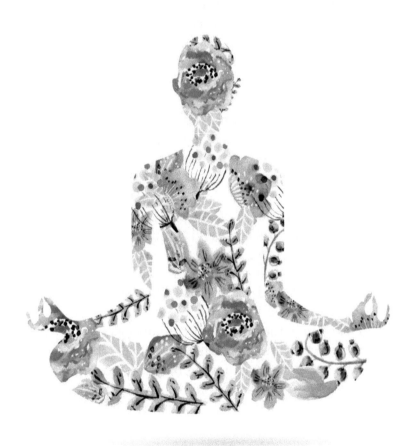

How to use this book?

This is a book of two halves.

The 'I AM' sections are my observations of events that have taken place in my personal and professional life that have shaped my beliefs about myself and the world around me. Ultimately these beliefs are part of an intrinsic internal dialogue, so loud that it has often left me unable to see or hear clearly and held me back from being authentically joyful. I have witnessed this in many of my clients too. I share what I have learned from these experiences and how our physical and energetic body is ultimately impacted.

In the 'YOU ARE' sections we get into the teachings of the five elements according to the yogic chakra system. Once we grasp the knowledge of the five elements and their associations to our physical and energetic body, we can then apply my rituals to each element inside our physical microcosm; the key to reflecting holistic harmony and balance back out to the macrocosm, the universe.

I have a request before you read on…. That you get ready to hang up your hang-ups, to peel away your facade and give yourself permission to expose your vulnerabilities. There is no weakness in this. If you can access this headspace you can, with a deliberate discipline apply my rituals to your everyday life with an open heart and mind that is full of space, ready to receive self-love and care willingly and give back to the universe abundantly. My wish is for you to take one piece of healthy inspiration from this small interpretation of 'what I think life is all about' and thencause that in your own life.

I AM great – believe it or not

*'Never underestimate the power of
dreams and the influence of the
human spirit. We are all the same
in this notion: The potential for
greatness lives within each of us.'*

Wilma Rudolph

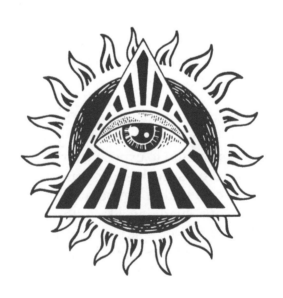

Getting back to the silent, suffering superhero. Have you ever been faced with a moment in your life, 'that moment' you've been waiting for - the chance to really express your voice?

Perhaps in that moment of enthusiasm and excitement, when you have plucked up the courage to express your thoughts or ideas in an area of your life, you are not received well. Your expectations of the outcome are shut down and pushed aside. It appears your idea or opinion isn't valid. You are faced with resignation. Your peers or superiors might laugh you off. 'You think this is a joke'? You ask yourself as you laugh with them to avoid awkwardness. God forbid people see a glimmer of frustration or anger in you. You could lose your job, that relationship, or the clear perception your family, friends and colleagues have of you. You fear you might be talked about in 'that' group, club or workplace if you pursue any communication remotely out of the box. The non-threatening approach is nicer and more friendly. You are the one who sticks to saying 'yes', even if you don't really mean 'yes'; the one who is willing to help and go along with others.

While you do this to be safe, you begin to doubt yourself-deeply and for a long time. You begin to question your sense of worth. 'Perhaps they are right. Maybe my contribution isn't valid'? In that small moment of internal turmoil, you might find yourself acting in a similar way to the example below...

You may unconsciously or consciously begin to re-affirm that you are not being heard and believe that your ideas and views are probably not good enough. You may then create a reason why, to justify the conclusion you have come up with. By acting this way, you don't have to

21

explain yourself to anyone, you save yours and everyone else's time and get on with your routine again. You keep pressing through life with hope and optimism that your contribution will be worth something eventually, one day or maybe you'll never get your chance, that is what you are agreeing to.

In this mindset you become engulfed in hopelessness and powerlessness, and that's it. That is your loop, your behaviour to this kind of situation and probably many other scenarios. You will remain in constant hopeless intention and never in action. The moment you become an intentional person who has no intention of taking action, you will become that very nice, uninspiring person who never gets anything complete in their life. Congratulations. You have good intentions. Do you feel better about yourself now? Until next time when the same pattern repeats itself and you experience the same circumstance and feelings. Perhaps you even have a nervous physiological response in your body that you start to get familiar with? It is worse the next time, so you gradually adapt and manage your bodily reactions with strategies, more reinforcements and excuses.

I have experienced this way; I have worked with many clients that can relate to this when they finally confront themselves. This inaction and self-defeat are a major contribution to repeated human suffering and separation in the modern world, keeping us small. I no longer buy into it.

Instead, when faced with these small yet significant challenges in our life we must re-program our default dialogue and create new and empowering actions for ourselves. For example, in that moment of recognition it is the exact moment to take yourself off to a quiet place. A meeting room, a bedroom, a corridor or even a toilet cubicle if necessary, and get a grip of yourself. Take all those emotions of frustration, humiliation, anger, resentment, hurt to name a few and channel them into focus, determination, productivity and composure. To recognise that your body and your energy is the hub of creative force and power, is the moment you become free of being a misused ego machine. The ego feeds off quick-fix habits that will only ever keep your head above water and your soul dampened down. The time is now - get to work and make a plan for your greatness to be heard!

'So, what's the magic?' you ask.

One way we master the chaos of the intellectual mind is by exploring our dirt! The gritty, layers that have been smeared across our soul; our light. This takes commitment and trust in our physical and energetic bodies; a spiritual investigation; and the unravelling of the old belief systems we are so loyally attached to.

When we start on this journey, we begin to constructively channel our findings with a clearer view and direct this cleaner self into our work arena, community, business and our personal space. We might find that our self-development was born in one place and then trickles through to many other facets that make up our life. Then, we must breathe, and be humble enough to give our newfound knowledge and wisdom away. Yes, that's right. Give it away. This may seem absurd. We spend our life doing things for 'I'.

'I' is the only thing we think we really have. Even when we are doing something for someone else it is quite easy to trace this back to the 'I'. 'I' becomes the centre of the universe. 'I' is the ego. The idea that we are separate or superior to nature's law. 'I' is arrogant at times. 'I' is hostile when it suits and holds its knowledge too close to its chest. 'I' is smug. YOU and WE are not 'I'.

We are nature. Holistic in form and vibration. Just another living organism passing through the cyclic patterns of life. Day by day, through winter, spring, summer and autumn, we are all in this together. The problem we have most of the time is lack of trust in this universal law, lack of trust in nature's truth. We learn to disassociate from our natural world and go on a material quest that is all about 'I and my life'.

The quest for material success, wealth and achievements fall under the law of economics. A way that is subtly drummed into us from an early age. If we enrol solely in the law of economics, there will always be a void and we will fundamentally always be willing or resentful servants but servants to money none the less. If at any moment along our way we get a mere glimpse of our internal spark of power, therein lies the opportunity to explore it. When we start cleaning up our junk and start seeing our own spark get bigger, we can then understand true compassion, an interconnection between us all. When we come to terms with the idea that we are individually unique but collectively the same, we see that we are all one. When this ancient wisdom is applied to our modern lifestyles miraculous shifts in consciousness can take place. We learn that we are not unique, yet we can still live a wonderful existence. Yet most of us unknowingly turn a blind eye to our profound intuitive intelligence.

I say this with conviction - after spending nearly my entire life working on my anxiety, I have accessed the place where there is freedom from judgment and suffering. This said, it is a daily practice, but it doesn't have to be an intense one. Once we meet and get to know our internal spark we can master our head brain and become detached from 'I'. We can let go of mental worry even when we experience the physiological feelings of nervousness and anxiety.

Having spent a big part of my life working out ways to survive, developing techniques and strategies to get by, working through fleeting emotions, moving forward with passion and purpose, I have learned this…From our birthright of being blissful come several storms. Through surviving the storms, we form our identity and our ego. Through a rising ego come several breakdowns and breakthroughs. When we shift ourselves from the internal dialogue and the mind, we can re- attune to universal awareness through conscious unravelling of our body's physical and esoteric layers. We re-discover our bliss and become a torch of greatness once again.

I AM mother

*'Rise goddess, rise and meet this day.
Child of the earth and the
stars, the heartbeat of the
universe is within you. So
breathe. Breathe and let the
winds of your spirit guide.
Relieve your shoulders of the burdens.
You are meant to fly.'*

S.C Lourie

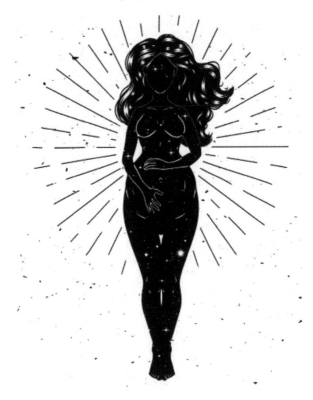

How did I get to this point in my life? Before, I always had something to look forward to. Something so significant to work for and talk about with friends. From the small occasions that fill up the diary to the big wish list; the life goals to achieve. I achieved lots. I always had a sense of excitement. A sense that 'things were yet to come'. I had my whole life ahead of me. That was before. When it was all about me. When I had all the time in the world and didn't know it. When lie -ins meant 11 am. When I depended so much on an alarm clock. When feeling tired was the equivalent to one little yawn on the scale of what that means today.

It hasn't been about me for years. Who is 'me' anyway? Just a little human being walking through life with lots of stories and experiences under her belt. A daughter, sister, friend, colleague, wife and now…mother. Yet, for some reason, the latter doesn't come under the 'me' category. 'Mother' has never felt like it belonged in that identity list. It has always felt separate to 'me'. Like she was a completely new person who I didn't know before but was somehow an intrinsic part of me. I was just experiencing the physical impact that comes from growing and creating children in my womb. It has taken *me* years after having my first child to get to know *her* - 'Mother'. It was life changing, hard and confusing.

For a while I believed it was stopping me from getting back to 'me'. This internal dialogue had to shift, or I would be going down a path of resistance, moaning and suffering for the rest of my life. I was seeing everything as a struggle and resigning myself to being unempowered - just 'getting on' with life. I was so attached to my old self and an idea of who she was and what she hadn't yet accomplished that I was ironically holding myself back from my growth as a mother. Achieving very little and knowing I wasn't at my best. I was exhausted with anxiety. Witnessing so much 'comparison-itis' around me.

Then there was a significant moment where I was stopped in my tracks. A moment where I decided that I didn't want to just 'get on' in life anymore. Getting on was my idea of hell. So, I surrendered. I chose to change my story. I chose to smash through the walls and obstacles, then, when I realised that way was a bit too aggressive and only caused more upheaval, I created my daily rituals. I nearly forgot for a moment there, that I had acquired a toolbox of holistic knowledge over years and now was the time that I needed them the most. I began PRACTICING and adapting my rituals to fit in with my lifestyle until it became an integral part of my life. This self-care work aided me to reign my energy back into my physical body and away from my chaotic head.

I made a verbal commitment directly into the mirror one day, staring at myself. I made a pledge to a handful of my bigger life goals and quietly kept them in the back of my mind, in my 'life goals commitment box'. I also wrote them down and put the note in my jewellery box so I could refer to it whenever I needed a reminder. I gave these dreams a rightful place so that I no longer obsessed over what I 'couldn't' do now that I was a mother. This made some space in my mind to focus on the smaller, achievable plans and daily duties. This space was the key component which gave me the freedom to function in a practical way. I could now take small daily actions and complete projects and duties without feeling overwhelmed.

This enabled me to learn the skill of flowing through pain, checking in with all the huge, unrealistic expectations I set myself and learning to embody each moment with my children, exactly as it was; chaotic or calm and without resistance.

'Mother' energy is within all of us. It is symbolic of the embodiment of feminine energy and all creative force within us. Men and women need to discover her, respect her and create her within. In my experience and practice, mother earth energy is the umbrella under which all the other labels reside, staying protected from whatever the weather chooses to be that day.

Come rain, storm or sunshine, mother takes the battering of life with a pinch of salt as long as she sticks to her *ground* rules; her baseline with which she resets and checks in to every day. It is essential for her to be rooted and resilient so that *water* can flow freely off her back. It is necessary for mother to bask in the *sun's energy* when she gets the chance, or she risks premature rusting. Mother will no doubt flip inside out in the *wind,* bending and bowing. However, mother does not break. She no longer relates to the limitations of the physical world. *She is the space holder, the joy spark, the facilitator* for herself, her family, her community, her world; to expand and grow in whatever way she chooses to create. As long as she/they always remain in the practice of authentic creation, constantly learning to re-form and re-emerge; re-creating in life is the sheer magic of life. Whether this be physically birthing a child, conceiving a business idea, seeing a life goal or project grow and evolve; discovering and channeling this innate feminine energy is where our personal power and inspiration is stored.

With this new perspective, 'mother' is suddenly more powerful and brave than she ever imagined. She is a force of nature. She is more than the elements combined and therefore mother is the creator of her own greatness - undeniably worthy of eminence, with no need to justify why and how she does 'being great'. She is stillness, movement and power all rolled into the cyclic rhythms of life. She is the shining light within us all.

I AM too little of this and too much of that...

*'Not being heard is no
reason for silence'*

Victor Hugo

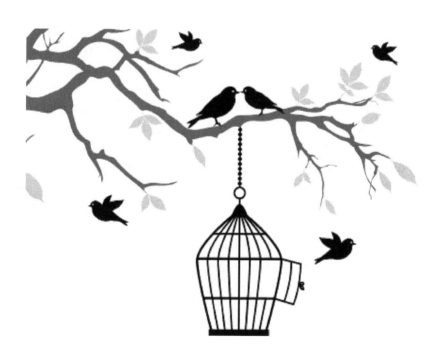

As a little girl I was always intuitive. Being the youngest of three I became an observer by default. Sensitive and reactive yet drawn to expressing myself through singing, writing, performance, movement and art. Needing to be heard no doubt! This is where I came alive. I still do, but from a very different vibration now. Back then I always felt a huge amount of shame for being 'too sensitive', 'too dramatic' or 'too deep' as people have told me I am. I always felt like I was doing something wrong if I cared or showed too much interest in other people. 'Too nosey' was another one. A sense that people got uncomfortable when I spoke truthfully, shared from the heart and had a genuine interest in what others were really thinking underneath the surface.

As I was growing up I was loud and chattery and never really taken seriously. My words were laughed off when in fact, I was serious about being heard and frustrated that I seemed to be getting smaller and smaller as I wanted to share my voice more and more. So, I learned to shut up and be quiet. I felt so odd and out of place and certainly not like others. Which is why I became so fascinated with the mind, self-exploration and the exposing of the raw truths in myself and encouraging others to reveal their truth too.

However, along the way I learned that people get very uncomfortable at the thought of their true thoughts and feelings being exposed. People don't want to be revealed for many reasons, the number one being through pure fear and lack of self-worth. This is no-one's fault. Encouraging myself to move out of the blame game was the first step for my own personal growth.

My view was that I came from a household where I never felt heard. This is my internal story. The one I have been telling myself most of my life and the one that has been vastly adapted by my clever mind to re-enforce my belief that I am never heard. This belief has formed the long-standing internal dialogue in my head that I am not worthy of being heard (lack of self-worth) and I am too scared to have a voice (fear of true expression). This is one of my many stories about myself. Stories that we as humans naturally create after stress and trauma, then cleverly and with the instinct of our primitive brain, hold on to so tightly to make sure we don't fall into the traps of those stresses and traumas ever again.

These stories make up our script and the script is played out on repeat, sometimes for months and sometimes for many years. Except the stories are now miles apart from the facts or events that took place when we were stressed or experiencing trauma. We have become deluded from the actual factual events and live by our emotive and meaningful stories. Therefore, we prevent ourselves from being open to any other belief about what we are capable of as humans. For the most part, we sit tight and get as comfortable as possible and ride the roller-coaster journey of life until its end.

So, as a kid who thought she didn't get heard the most sensible thing to do was to sing my heart out for release or shout to the point of tears when I felt strongly about a situation. I was extremely frustrated. I did this for a long period of my childhood which caused a now obvious energetic imbalance in my body. There was a fluctuating pattern of overstimulation or depletion in my nervous system, especially in the throat and neck area (pharyngeal/cervical plexus) and the stomach area (solar/celiac plexus). This manifested into chronic neck and stomach tension and I believe pre-disposed me to the thyroiditis and silent acid reflux that I later suffered with. I was in a habitual, subconscious cycle which fuelled anxiety, caused upper chest breathing which created more anxiety, and so the cycle continued.

Adding insult to injury, I still actively manage old whiplash and backpain from incidents that have happened which inevitably induce weakness into the already fragile energy centres. I didn't know any of this back then! I had no idea that the mind and body were connected in this way. I had no idea about the law of attraction or the polarity theory which I will later discuss in chapter -YOU ARE matter and mind and chapter – YOU ARE a gift to yourself.

When I look back now, I see a confused girl seeking attention and truth. I see someone who was a bit 'slow' in formal learning settings which then became another belief in my mind -

'I am not good enough so I need to prove to everyone that I can do it as well as, if not better than them.'

I later learned that all my efforts in this area still didn't get me any closer to being seen or heard! (My original belief made from my single sided story). It only stoked my system into overdrive or underdrive. Are you still with me?

Nowadays, those gaps of seeking approval are slowly closing up as I stick more to the facts and the energetic intuition and less to wild imagination. The past doesn't exist, and the future doesn't yet exist. Therefore, the only thing left to do is be present, solid in the cold hard reality of living on this earth whilst simultaneously being the simple vessel for the wonders of life and experiences to pass through. In this reality my voice is much clearer and therefore I can make clearer choices, stick to my word and take constructive action from the choices I make.

Choosing to be at a place transcendent of my comfort zone and old belief system of needing to be accepted took training the mind and tuning the heart. How did I transform these old patterns of shouting loudly in order to be heard? By getting real.

Thoughts, feelings and physical sensations are always going to be there. The human body plays out its daily duties, cell by cell and system by system, constantly altering on a biochemical level to be in homeostasis and work together as one whole living and breathing vessel. We must have the utmost respect for our beautiful bodies for being our vehicles and giving us the ability to function in this way. The doubts and fears also show up daily in our internal dialogue. I no longer believe that we can change ourselves. As if, something is faulty that needs fixing or replacing. No. I now fully accept my worth. I am fully in-love with my truthful voice and equally my woes. I share myself authentically with the world despite all the made-up stuff that tries to get in the way. There will always be off days which come with being human, of course. This is why a self-care practice has become my life ritual and the very steady thing that has enabled me to fly with purpose and contribution.

The old life for me was thinking that to be considered as able and worthy I must say what people want to hear because no-one likes the truth. I must come face-to-face with an assessment, waiting for consent - but from whom? The invisible jury? Then I would need to report back to get my results on whether I did a good enough job of being 'me' or not.

This translates to feeling chained to authority and judgment which is all just an illusion; very low vibrational energy, trickery from the primitive survival brain whose job it is to keep us small and safe. As much as we still depend on our primitive brain, we also have an advanced brain, plus a gut brain and a heart brain. Our heart brain has approximately 40,000 neurotransmitters and sends more information to the brain than the brain does to the heart. The gut brain, arguably the brain that developed before our central nervous system, functions independently from the head brain, yet we intuitively know that our heart, gut and head are connected. Have you ever had your heart broken or had a gut feeling when you are nervous?

Because we are so governed by our cerebral intellect, we get easily distracted and ignore the other intelligence held in our body. If we want to attain balance in all areas of our life we need to explore and respect all areas of our body as equal and synergistic.

Do you resonate with this chapter?

Refer to chapter 'YOU ARE a gift to yourself – ELEMENT – Space' to discover more.

Trauma memory 1 -
I AM hateful

*'You use a glass mirror to see
your face; you use works of art
to see your soul'*

George Bernard Shaw

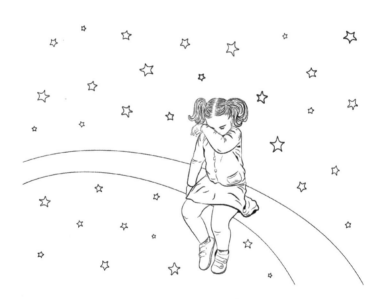

There are some crucial memories that stand out for me which I have been able to access through transformative training methods, science and holistic based therapy, such as cognitive behavioral therapy, cranio-sacral therapy and chakra balancing. By doing this and coming face-to-face with these memories I have been able to locate the moments when my negative internal dialogue took shape. I have used my memory to deeply heal the detrimental self-talk that has shaped much of how I viewed and acted in the world, and consequently, what the world has reflected back at me. Re-routing these patterns of negative self-talk and lack of direction has enabled me to see clearly and be confident in my choices.

I was just like the majority of three-year-olds, pottering about my day, curious about the adventures that my brothers were up to and in need of a lot of attention. Having said this, I was a perceptually happy child. I have the fondest memories of my childhood. I say perceptual because that is what it is. Everyone's perception is different. It is something that naturally changes as we age and gather more information for our brains to rationalise and process.

Along with all the subtle doubts I was storing up, in those early days I developed ways to stand my ground. I learned very early on that fighting for what I wanted was how things got done. With two older and confident brothers, my daily mission was to try and get ahead, listen out for vital information and never be caught out! I might have been slow in education, but I thought I was the best detective. My brothers were bigger and stronger than me, overall, very affectionate towards me but equally our brawls were gruesome.

Now, as I learn more about the human brain I see that these early experiences really have been the roots of major behavioral patterns that have been with me for a long time and played out in my body's memory and my adult life. Such as, feeling my muscles move into a heightened, contracted state when I think I am being confronted by my loved ones over who's right and who's wrong on a topic of conversation. The desperate need to be acknowledged by my loved ones and for them to validate my intelligence rather than see me as 'the little one' who can't know what she's talking about. There it is - my struggle, the suffering for what I want, the fight to be heard, and there is no freedom in this.

The night my mum drove me back home after my eye surgery we arrived into chaos and fear as we discovered we had been burgled. I still remember sitting on the kitchen counter with a big patch over my eye and crying out of the other eye as my dad stood on the outside of the house repairing our smashed kitchen window. I felt uncomfortable and sore, after having had a squint corrected which required my eyeball to be taken out of its socket and some muscles cut and sewn back together. Yet this wasn't at the forefront of my mind, having our house burgled was. It was one of the first times I felt unstable and scared. It was a very real distraction from my eye surgery and the condition I had lived with my whole life, which had never really been discussed.

My 'off' visual appearance was never really acknowledged and that always bothered me. My eye turned inwards and although the operation helped, I used to get double vision from time to time, I would often reach for things not knowing the accurate distance of the object and then drop whatever it was I was trying to grasp. The same for catching balls or playing hand to eye co-ordination games. So here was my reality back then - I wore big glasses and had thick auburn hair. I didn't feel 'pretty' and none of my close family and friends ever confirmed to me that my squint was still visible after the surgery, even though I could see it when I looked in the mirror and there is evidence of it in photographs. Whenever I used to bring it up I didn't get very far without being told I was silly and that there was nothing wrong with me. This wasn't true to me though, as much as those words 'there is nothing wrong' were spoken, I didn't feel right.

Then it was confirmed. Hooray! I wasn't going crazy, thinking that only I could see this definite truth and no-one else could. Except this confirmation over the mystery squint was given to me by the bullying I received in the playground. Every time I looked in the mirror, I could see something was 'wrong' which I translated as 'I AM not perfect'. This imperfection festered into years of hatred for my visual appearance and hatred for anyone who negatively commented on my imperfections. So much so, I would actively avoid those people in the playground or classroom for fear of being shown up and laughed at. I felt physical pain with every comment which inevitably fueled a deep lack of self-worth.

Do you resonate with this chapter?

Refer to chapter 'YOU ARE a gift to yourself – ELEMENT – Earth' to discover more.

Trauma memory 2 - I AM powerless

'Things are not always as they seem; the first appearance deceives many'

Phaedrus, written by Plato

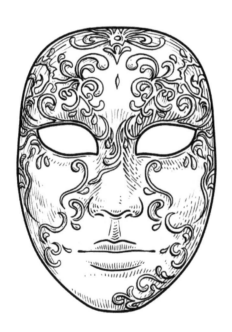

Back in my early years we had a couple of au-pairs sent to us from an agency. The last one, 'the horrible one' as my mother called her, was no match for our first Au-pair Karin 'the lovely one'. The horrible one was moody, irritated and didn't know how to handle a small child. She couldn't cope with the toddler tantrums and got to the point where she felt she had to restrain me so I wouldn't run around and cause chaos - as normal children do! My father returned home from work one afternoon to find a screaming; distressed child in the bathroom and tied to the bath taps. As he untied and comforted me, I didn't know at the time that I would be left confused over this for many years after.

I clearly remember being thrown in an old cot several times in our spare room with the door slammed in my face for what felt like hours. Again, to the point of hysteria. No-one came. I remember feeling trapped until finally the door opened, and I was whisked downstairs by the au pair just in time for my parents to come home and not suspect a thing. When I told my parents about this memory years later, they didn't think I would be able to remember that far back. It was only when they revealed the bath taps memory that things started to connect. This memory is vague in my mind but very real in my body. I am not sure what's worse. Experiencing a trauma that you remember clearly or being told of a trauma that you can't clearly recall yet feeling all the sensations of anxiety and sadness as you recollect it.

The 'horrible' au pair was sent back to Switzerland with my mum's designer shoes smuggled in her suitcase and was never to be seen again. And nothing more was said about that for years! Being so young, I found a way to survive those incidents. Yet that nervous residue stayed in my physical body for another 22 years before I ever looked at it and began healing through it. When the bath taps story was brought up at a family dinner one night, my parents recounted it with jovial contemplation, talking about the crazy au-pair who stole the shoes and tied me to the bath taps. It was in this moment that I was experiencing a very different, gut wrenching sensation. I was overcome with terror. As if my body had entered a 'recall' state and gone into some sort of shock. I began to feel the physical surges of panic, wondering what else might have happened to me all the other times that my parents weren't aware of and that I can't clearly remember.

This recollection sent me on one of my first forays into deep inquiry. Desperate to get the facts from my parents and make sense of it all. I knew that my body was relating to these events and trying to send me subtle communication, but I couldn't comprehend it in my logical brain. I grew increasingly frustrated. I began to convince myself that I grew up under some illusion; that my privileged childhood was disturbing.

Parallel to this recollection I began to study body therapy, starting with Ayurveda and Indian Head Massage and then onto advanced remedial body work, aromatherapy for stress and cranio-sacral therapy for trauma release.

I managed to scramble my way through the playground jungles, coming out of the other side at age 18 with many (what I call) 'mini traumas', a few mental scars, some physical ones and some weird anxiety quirks. Yet I felt that I was finally on the road to having it all figured out. I was free.

I found ways to manage anxiety and social awkwardness, ways to control my panic attacks in moments of discomfort or fear, strategies to manage my physical pain from injuries. I was so naïve. I had only become more tense, more controlling and more nervous as I got older and used to mask my suffering underneath a big smile. The result? Pretending and trying hard to hold it all together when in fact I was centre stage at my own circus. I had become the juggling clown, waiting for a whole lot of laughs which would help validate me and justify my existence. When I didn't get any reactions, I would talk myself into being not worthy of acknowledgment of my accomplishments. I had several bandages wrapped around me, cleverly disguised as reasons and excuses from shying away and avoiding my powerful authentic self.

Little did I know that these layers covering up my physical and emotional pain didn't realise that my clever body stores all the memories deep inside on a muscular, fascial, cellular level. Memories are not just stored in the brain where we can reason with them. When I discovered body therapy, energy healing, yoga and self-development I was embarking on a complete transformation and in for a true roller-coaster ride, not just for myself but for all my future clients as well.

Do you resonate with this chapter?

Refer to chapter 'YOU ARE a gift to yourself – ELEMENT – Fire' to discover more.

Trauma memory 3
I AM unloved

*'The course of true love
never did run smooth'*

William Shakespeare

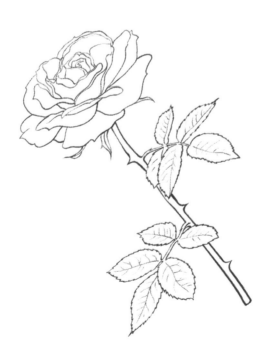

After my A-levels I couldn't wait to escape my little world of woes and dramas. I embarked on my first travelling adventure which in and around university turned into four epic and life changing tours, and eventually a huge part of my holistic work.

This was my first real taste of freedom and exposure to an alternative world to the one I had lived in my entire life; the first time I could use my voice and be heard! I was ecstatic.

Of course, when you are that high the inevitable is a big gut-wrenching low at some point. This was during a time when I had no awareness of a happy, balanced mid-point. I was governed by my emotions and external influences. Having said this, to be 'that' person who rides on her emotions, and changes direction like the wind, the ramifications of being dumped by your first love, on a riverboat, in the middle of the thick amazon jungle sounds too far fetched to be real. It was real though. That did happen, but I couldn't acknowledge or believe it for a long time. The drama was too much to bear, the emotions were too extreme.

This event became one of my most extreme internal stories. I would use it to justify my belief that no-one could ever love me and, in turn, that no one could ever be trusted, not even those closest to me. That day I didn't know whether to jump in the river that was full of piranha's or push him in instead! Of course, I did neither. It was the first time I felt numb and resigned to my reality. There was no amount of controlling or convincing that was going to change this reality. That day, I also swam with pink dolphins and fished for piranha which we cooked on the campfire that night. I had surprisingly lost my appetite for those man-eating fish by then! These were once in a lifetime moments, riddled with a heaviness. The injustice I felt was raging in me. The fact that I would have to live with these memories for the rest of my life knowing that they were born out of the most shattering circumstances. It wasn't meant to be this way. This wasn't how I had imagined my trip around the world. I wasn't supposed to be left sad, rejected and heart broken. I couldn't come to terms with that for a long time. I remained on our group tour of South America for two more weeks. Making more incredible memories with a person I was never going to be able to recount them with. Knowing that when all this was over and we got out of the forest and back into the city we would be logistically free to go our separate ways.

We went on an anaconda hunt through the pampas. We cycled down the worlds most dangerous road in Bolivia, we toured across the salt flats for days, we partied in Rio and kayaked around Isla Grande. I had so many incredible adventures and memories with the 'ex that dumped me on the riverboat'. I had to carry on and travel through town and country until I could get to a computer, email my friends who were travelling around the same time and arrange to meet them, finally parting ways with him.

Aside from the anger and deep sadness that had been creeping over me for weeks, I didn't realise how much resentment was festering inside. Not just from this unfortunate situation but from all the other unjust events in my past. I began to live wild and recklessly because I was determined not to let this incident ruin my nomadic adventures. The temporary result of this was that I had the time of my life for my remaining time as a *gringo*. I decided to be completely carefree even though I profoundly cared.

The drama and trauma continued as my travels did. In Cambodia, my friend and I were evacuated from our hotel in the middle of the night when a fire broke out. We were locked on an overnight bus in Vietnam with our passports confiscated and, I was hospitalized when my drink was spiked with elephant tranquilizer! These traumas seemed so unreal that I somehow managed to play them down and laugh about them. As if they were just part and parcel of travelling and choosing to live on the edge. Inside, I was in complete survival mode with high functioning anxiety for years to come. The hurt, let down and panic wouldn't be addressed for years. I simply needed a story to hold onto to explain and rationalise what had happened to me. I was the victim and this manifested in my body in the form of irritation and years of inflamed adult acne and panic attacks. I had resigned myself. My nervous system was shot to pieces and this constant anxiety wasn't sustainable.

The universe had been sending me signs that I either wasn't seeing or hearing or was simply ignoring. Up until that point in my life I was volcanic. Slowly bubbling away, but somewhat dormant. Finally, I felt as though the universe had enough and ultimately rocketed me out of my comfort zone for good on the 'amazon jungle day' as I call it. That wretched day was the beginning of my transition from girl to woman.

Do you resonate with this chapter?

Refer to chapter 'YOU ARE a gift to yourself – ELEMENT – Air' to discover more.

Trauma memory 4 –
I AM torn

'Pain is inevitable,
suffering is optional'

Buddhist proverb

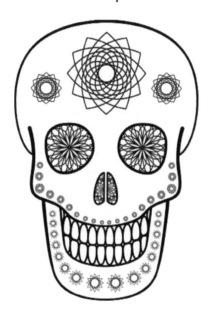

A long-term boyfriend, the international lifestyle, the yogic philosophy; getting married and having kids were the next things on the 'to do' list. Although I wasn't the sort of person who wanted to look good and keep up with the Jones's, I was unconsciously falling back into place, doing all the things that you do to adhere to society's order. I was conditioned and acting like I wasn't conditioned. I hated being conventional and had seen a much bigger world than the comfortable one I had grown up in, yet I was programmed to follow suit. and that's what I did.

At the start of 2014 something remarkable happened to me. I died, metaphorically but nearly quite literally. My 30 years of life as I knew it became irrelevant that day. I was faced with a new identity, a new body, a new perspective and a new baby. If my exact birthing experience had taken place 60 years earlier the likelihood of me and my baby surviving were very small. I was physically and metaphysically shut tight! I was ashamed that I – the yogi, the energy worker, the therapist, the vegetarian could not give birth the way that nature intended in my first pregnancy.

I felt violated by the countless examinations I had undergone and, to top it off, my final labouring hours were spent hooked up to a machine with the surgeons head between my legs trying to insert pulse pads and a catheter tube which later got caught on the hospital bed guard as they transferred me to the operating table. As if contractions weren't painful enough, according to my husband, the scream that came out of me sounded like I was being murdered. I was then given a spinal block with a fear of paralysis. This wasn't going down well.

At the time of my first pregnancy I had become accustomed to jet-setting around the world for work. I had the best job, in an industry that I loved and had worked hard in. I got to travel far and wide, stay in luxury spa hotels and teach therapists yoga, glorious healing treatments and the wonders of natural skincare products. I was living the dream. Although on my days off I would work on admin until the early hours of the morning to play catch-up for being in practical training all day, I still got the chance to mosey around a tropical Maldivian island or visit a market in Vietnam. I saw sacred temples in Bali and hopped on boat trips around the Golden Gate bridge or the Everglades to spot some alligators.

Back to the labour ward and this was not the same life. My incense never left my hospital bag. My aromatherapy oils and yogic mantra music didn't get a look in. My labour experience was the first thing that was out of my control in a very long time. You see, I had engineered my life to avoid any more pain and strive for purity and perfection. It got to a point when I had to give up control. This was forced on me when the anaesthetist told me we had run out of time, my baby was in distress as was I having a major panic attack like never before. This was my experience of sheer terror. He simply had to insert that needle into my spine. There was no turning back.

What will be will be; yet my brain could not rationalise this process as I entered a trauma survival state and began to shut down.

I gave birth to my wonderful son via c-section that day. I was also new-born. A new-born mother. What a blessing, I should be so grateful, and I was. I was also traumatised, shocked, in immense pain post-surgery, injecting myself with anticoagulants for the next week and sleep deprived before I even got my mother game on!

The following two years was a blur. I felt powerless and weak, unable to take full ownership of my responsibilities as a mother. I was so in love with my baby and did everything the right and best way I knew how. There were many significant 'present' moments with my son in those early days but for the most part I was riddled with guilt, worry or a deep sense of...

'what if we had died that day? How should I be doing parenting better?'

A thick haze sat over my head. We were so lucky to be alive, but I couldn't feel alive for a long time. Being told by nearly every mother I encountered that 'guilt' will become a normal emotion after having children raised huge alarm bells and a disturbed feeling in me. Surely this isn't how motherhood should feel?

After having my first child my life got so heavy with anxiety and shock. My experience of going back to work and appearing to have it all together as a return to work mum in a job I loved just didn't feel good for me anymore. My job title got bigger, my paycheck got bigger and I grew more conflicted. It didn't feel like I had it all. It felt awful. I felt I had been tricked into this 'to do' game without knowing all the facts and consequences that come with being a parent.

Every day I would wake up guilty to be leaving my baby at the child minders, yet relish having a cup of coffee with a work colleague and talking to an adult. I would then forget about my child for three hours whilst immersed in my to do list, only ever achieving half of every job at a time. Then, being in a mad rush to get one task completed to a deadline and not feeling it was my best work. Then wondering what my tiny baby was up to. Had I missed anything? Was the child minder following his little routine properly? I was riddled with worry. All the while working in a wellness and spa industry, where it was my job to promote health, happiness and a luxury modern lifestyle. Things weren't in alignment at all. I was totally out of whack. After the delusion of maternity leave which I thought was the thing I had always wanted - a big, glorified holiday, I realised that life doesn't get 'better' after having a kid, it gets busier, more stressful, more demanding than ever before. I was searching for better all the time and better got the best of me. After experiencing the most physical pain I had ever encountered in my life I couldn't see the rich colours and beautiful chaos that a baby brings. Instead my pain grew, in my head, into suffering.

On the one hand, my child brought me sheer joy. Cuddling him, watching him potter around, singing sweetly, watching him sleep – it's true love. Yet, what follows this bliss is the overwhelming sense of duty and responsibility. I wanted to ensure that he got the best chance in this life yet spent my time worrying that he was not. I wanted him to always preserve his bliss, but I also needed to make sure he was fed, watered, educated and exactly where he was meant to be according to the mad family schedule.

I wasn't at ease with this life. I had spent years being away from 'normal' and then found myself deep in the undergrowth of a family existence, battling with my desires vs. my new duties. What just happened?

Do you resonate with this chapter?

Refer to chapter 'YOU ARE a gift to yourself – ELEMENT – Water' to discover more.

&

I AM Born

'Failure is only a perception born from a seed of doubt. To be released from failure is to trust that you are worthy of love'

Carly Chamberlain

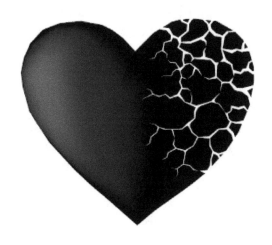

At the start of November 2016, I died…again. This time, I was sitting at my kitchen table staring out of the window. I had my lovely toddler pottering around my feet and I was seven weeks pregnant. Still doing my dream job, in senior management, but the most miserable I have ever felt in my working life. I was doing a full-time job in three to four days a week. I was on emails at night trying to catch up and stay on top of deadlines, there was a vile, passive-aggressive work colleague breathing down my neck and my life was not in-line with the life I had in mind. That day, I got in the car to go on a long weekend away, a much needed rest whilst the grandparents took the reins. A lorry drove into the passenger side of my car several times with my son in the back seat, spinning us full circle until we were forced onto the hard shoulder. I had smashed glass in my mouth as I launched back to unclip my son from his seat. The car was smoking, I couldn't open the door as it was smashed in. I eventually found us sitting on the side of the motorway curled in a ball, as if my brain had checked out momentarily whilst my body went through the motions of getting us to safety. We just sat, waiting for someone to help us as I feared for my unborn baby's life and the damage this might do to my son.

The paramedics checked us over and said we were ok. Lucky to be alive. Of course, they had seen much worse. My boy wasn't injured externally, I had an early foetal scan and everything was fine with the pregnancy. It was all just fine, and everything was ok. Everyone around me was being positive and repeatedly saying 'you are so lucky it didn't go the other way'. But I wasn't fine. I wasn't ok. None of this made me feel relieved or better. My internal state was even worse now than before I got in the car that morning. In the weeks following the accident, my severe whiplash prevented me from picking up the kettle without feeling like I was going to drop it. I couldn't stand up without feeling dizzy and, to this day I have to talk myself into a rational space before we get on a motorway.

I was finally diagnosed with chronic post-traumatic stress syndrome and mild depression. I resigned from my job, had months of cognitive behavioural therapy, remedial massage rehab and cranio-sacral therapy for both my son and I. I STOPPED everything in order to surrender and accept healing and recovery. If I wanted my pregnancy to be safe and healthy and if I wanted to transform the life I found myself in, all I knew is that this life as I had been living it needed to shift.

Being willing to receive support and healing was the biggest obstacle I faced. I had always been the facilitator, the educator and therapist who takes care of everyone else, yet now, the therapist needed therapy! Having to surrender to receive was a whole new domain for me. I needed my family and friends, I welcomed the help much easier with my second birth than my first. Everything that was important to me from my life before children became secondary during this time. I accepted that becoming a mother was not just the next thing that I was supposed to do. It impacted every part of my life and now their lives. That's right. It wasn't all about me anymore and when I really got this, my maternal nature was finally ignited.

After several months of recuperation and the welcoming of our new baby to the family, my post-natal creative energy rose up and I gave birth to something new. My rituals. Self-care like never before. I returned to my holistic toolbox again and this time I meant business. And so, my wellness business sprouted up like a little seedling that had been germinating under the mud for years. Having a focus that I believed in gave me strength and held me up in those daily, stolen moments. Being kind to myself and releasing all expectation of perfection was the biggest relief. In return, my personal health and my wellness business grew.

I had been an advocate of health and wellness for so long, but I realised that I hadn't been nurturing myself in a loving way at all. I was functioning in a way that involved learning my craft, developing it and being of service to others whilst having no boundaries and ignoring my own fundamental needs. My lifestyle balance was completely out of kilter up until that point. As much as the dream career was a period filled with wonderful experiences and professional and personal development, I was still working 14-hour days with no consistent time off. If I worked harder, maybe I would be more successful? Nope. Not anymore. Not if it compromised my integrity, my values and most importantly my health (mind, body and soul) and family balance. I felt as though I had blinked and suddenly I was sitting with my two innocent children by my side watching them grow, watching them learn and process their surroundings. I started to relate to them more as I spent more time with them. I gave myself the moments to explore how their little lives were shaping out. Then I realised something remarkable. Every move I make and word I speak is taken on by them. They are always watching me. Every bad day, good day, mood swing, singing in the car moment, and argument, is a piece of information that they will process, and a feeling they will retain - unconsciously or consciously.

I asked myself, who do I want to be for them? I decided it was time to up my game in life.

I was determined not to reach the levels of anxiety I had done previously, which meant I needed to let all the old dirt and concerns go so that I could trust the signals being sent from the universe and trust myself - inside and out. This action enabled me to make powerful choices about what I wanted for my life, rather than operating from a fear and servant mentality.

Fear of losing a job, fear of not having enough money, fear of losing my reputation in an industry I love because I chose to take a breath and reflect. Fear of having a gap on the C.V which would raise questions in future job prospects. All these illusions were a very clear reflection of being chained to fear and subsequently depriving myself of great time freedom and success. Having a break and creating something new was nothing to fear. Stopping was nothing to be scared of. I began to experience a power within me to choose who I wanted to work with, choose my service value and have it aligned with my fundamental values.

I started to see growth in all areas of life, not just work. An ease in the way I was being for myself and others. Even when I was doubting this newfound approach to my work/family life and tempted to apply for that big job when we were worried about finances, I was reminded of this new power within me. So much so, that the idea of working in a job that wasn't in tune with my passions and beliefs eventually became an alien concept to me. Not having to compromise on a salary or a title, not having to sell myself as something inauthentic. I realised I could build a life that I believed in. I could build transparent healthy relationships, new working partnerships, continue to train and evolve my craft, expand my knowledge of Ayurveda and get back onto my yoga mat and do this without ever compromising on my core values or my precious time. This was liberation and ultimate fulfillment.

As for my family, wanting to desperately be a perfect mother and having such a lack of vital energy, disabled my internal eye. I couldn't see past all the things 'I had to do' to survive.

Surely all my training would give me the answers. I always have the right solutions! But after recovering from our car accident and making the shifts in my life, I was left with this beautiful stillness around me. It was in this still space, I learned all the things it takes to just 'be'. Much like meditation yet not needing to go away somewhere to meditate. Simply being in every moment, whatever the chore, or demand. In this newfound speechless space there is clarity and peace. A place where I learned to be fun and loving for my children. A place where judgment doesn't exist, pressure to be something you are not isn't there. The place where my little humans can just be loved, the place where I can be a blank canvas for them rather than try to paint my picture of who I want them to be. They will for sure have their own anxieties, traumas and fears in life. I don't have a microscope to see how they will process their experiences; however, I can now see that by ultimately 'being' with them, tuning into the present, instead of always 'doing' with them, thinking back or ahead, I can be totally selfless and still feel full; and in those off days that will inevitably be more of a challenge than others, I have the tools to find that balance between giving my energy to them, and taking responsibility of my own self-care without my cup feeling empty as it did before.

As we all know, speaking our intentions is far easier than acting on them. So, what next? This is my biggest question since having my children. My life with children has been my biggest growth. Before, I thought life was busy and that I knew it all. Nowadays every minute of my time is accounted for and I spend my days setting reminders on my phone. Parents are always needed and always busy. How do we juggle the needs and get all our tasks achieved? Time can be our greatest ally or our greatest enemy. Kids don't have this conundrum because they live in the moment. They will either start something and finish it or start something, drop it and move onto the next. With no regret, no second thought. It is what it is, and they do what they do and seem much happier for it. They only see what is in front of them. It is when we start to pressure them with the concept of time that things can feel out of control for us and upset them. It is safe to say my children have been my teachers in the lessons of action, but the question is how we become masters of time in order to balance our family's needs and, crucially, our own self-care.

Time has become everything and nothing to me. Learning to be truly present to what is going on in the physical body, the energy body (mind and emotions) and the soul doesn't involve clock watching. This is something much more subtle. To connect with time effectiveness in this way is to authentically embody 'the pause in time', even when things are moving extremely fast in everyday life. Visualising myself as a calm vessel inside a storm. This requires commitment but it does not have to be another thing on the to do list which takes up time and causes stress. It is not a feeling; it is a decisive commitment to being in alignment with self-care and self-power.

We still need to get places 'on time', so to move from A to B with more ease, requires planning and being in alignment with our needs and taking action to manage our needs. Being acutely aware of the messages we are receiving from our body, rather than neglecting them and then finding ourselves running around chasing our tails, requires doing what we say we are going to do and moving our intentions into actions.

Taking responsibility for time is the key to thriving in every moment whether it be good or bad. Learning a level of self-respect that enables you to be the creator of your time management, rather than existing on the receiving end, requires you to observe your outside self. Watching yourself from a bird's eye view.

What do you look like from up there? Always rushing around, panicking, being late and blaming it on someone or something else. 'The kids wouldn't put their shoes on in time'. 'The kids didn't finish their breakfast in time'. 'This happened and that happened'. To be unattached from time is the access to time success.

I AM letting go

'Life is what happens to you while you're busy making other plans.'

John Lennon

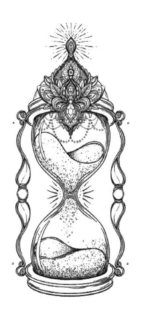

Death remains a sensitive topic of conversation. Almost a taboo subject that deserves so much more attention than it gets. Let us just face it! Let's look death in the face so that we can grasp the very real fact that one minute there is a living and breathing entity and the next minute there is a sack of potatoes, stuffed with chemical preservatives, made – up to resemble the person they once were but now squashed into a coffin. That is death. You may think 'This is so depressing'. Yes, it is. It is so sad, weird, and unfair. When we or someone we know experiences a death, we might meet that long-lost relative at the funeral and stick to the same 'safe' dialogue: 'I am so sorry for your loss'; 'I hope the day goes as best as it can'; 'It's so lovely to see you again, even though it's on this sad occasion'; 'so-and-so sends their condolences'. Although the intention is kind, I can't help but feel that we are forever treading on eggshells - we are so uncomfortable and in fear of upsetting the already upset! Then of course we might say the classic line - 'how are you?', then pause and cringe because we both know that they are not good at all having just lost their loved one.

I have lost so many loved ones, been close to death myself and worked with clients who come to me deeply grieving over someone or something they have lost. When I have been in treatment with my client's and work energetically, especially over their upper back and chest, (their heart centre) I witness incredible physical responses. If they are holding onto some form of loss and then have a breakthrough in 'letting go' I physically see this happening for them. An increase in rapid breathing followed by a deep sigh of relief; an emotional outburst; a verbal outcry; a hysterical response; a resistance which forces them to move or pause the treatment to go to the bathroom. It's fascinating! There loss may not necessarily be from dying. Other forms of loss include divorce or separation; a miscarriage or stillbirth; a surgical removal or repair; a relocation; a friendship breaking down or leaving a workplace after a long period of time. This has led me to inquire deeply into the behaviour and emotions associated with grief, and of course those fundamental questions about life and what it's all about.

If there is any place that highlights one's reaction to loss, it is at a funeral service. I have been to many funerals and there has been a consistent realisation every single time. As the religious cleric or celebrant shares reassuring words from either their chosen holy book or philosophy, there is a sense of sombre resignation amongst the majority. Some who are committed to their faith, find support and hope. Others stay numb, perhaps having no chosen faith or belief in religion and unable to rationalise it in their brain. The ones who are engulfed by their emotions which they feel they should not reveal in public. Rarer still, the ones who fully express their emotions, releasing them and moving through the pain. On the whole, most of us desperately try to contain our grief and sadness. This pain can be felt in the physical body and keeping it there will only prolong the grieving and healing process.

Bereavement and grieving can, for some, last a lifetime: from the moment you know you are going to lose something or someone close to you to long after they are gone. Although I may be stating the obvious, what I don't think we acknowledge enough is that we collectively have exactly the same feelings as everyone else. Anger, regret, deep sadness, confusion, resent, the list goes on. These are human feelings. So, if we all feel the same, why do we often find it so hard to share these emotions with others as a way of talking through our grief? Why is it so difficult to take action, to heal rather than wait for 'things to pass'? 'Letting things pass' is like saying, I am just going to let all this pain sink deeper and deeper into my cells, building more and more residue into my energetic field until I am swamped with what becomes unconscious grief and suffering and ultimately dis-ease.

Releasing and expressing our emotions (without being consumed by them as an unhealthy habit) is a great reminder to be gentle on ourselves. Although we know that the power of our thoughts can move our feelings in different directions such as resistance, we must also find a means of accepting and flowing through these natural emotions during periods of sadness and grief.

We are all on a pathway to discovering ourselves, whether we like it or not. We can turn our back on it, brush things under the rug for as long as we want, but when the end is near I believe we all have to face ourselves; our existence; our purpose; and ask ...Have I really contributed to the world as best as I could have?

When I was 17 - I lost my closest grandma. This was my first raw experience of grief. My grandad died when I was seven and I only remember a few brain memories of the experience rather than the physical pain in my heart and guts that overwhelmed me when my grandma died. Three weeks after she passed, I lost my other grandparents – who miraculously died on the same day. I say miraculously because in amongst all the unfathomable sadness I felt around that time I could only rationalise their passing as a pure miracle. How they managed to pop their clogs on the same day is still a mystery to me. Within all the confusion and pain, there was no other way to explain the experience other than utterly wondrous and astonishing. Yes, they were 91 and 93, yes, they had long, hard lives and their time was up. I ask my relatives now about their take on the story, as I spent some time telling my version and doubting myself that it was even true. I am still in awe of it to this day.

My grandad died at home and two hours later my grandma died in the hospital where she was recovering. Nobody notified her of her husband's passing as it was the early hours of the morning, she just slipped away or as I believe, followed her soul mate into the ether. They had been together for over 60 years with only a handful of days apart from each other. They had a double funeral, and this was my first experience of a miracle - in life and death. Others would say this is simple co-incidence. In response I say this…

Since those deaths I had a few years break from funerals and bereavement. I clung onto my cathartic story of my grandparents all dying within three weeks of each other as a way of reassurance that death wasn't always an unkind or unfair experience. Then it felt like, out of nowhere, one close relative or friend after another was leaving us every year. This phase went on for nine years. For a time, I became obsessed with counting how many had gone, still in disbelief that they were no longer with us. It's still a concept that most of us can't comprehend and it raises the biggest questions of all: Where do we go? What is this all about? Is there a heaven or an afterlife?

I became completely unsurprised on hearing about the next one 'kicking the bucket'. I felt desensitized and almost had an expectation of news of another death in our family. Then, the funeral day would come and I'd be overwhelmed with emotions every single time, forcing myself to find a distraction to control or suppress my tears (yes, I was that one!) - focusing on that little cherub painted on the ceiling to help me stop sobbing.

Death never gets easier for me. But one thing is clear in all my experiences. The departed are always referred to as returning to space/ ether as the physical body returns to the earth or fire spirit. This re-confirms that we are simply living organisms, part of nature's cycle. Yes, we have brains and a beating heart. Yes, we have intuition, consciousness and spirit. Yet, reminding ourselves that we are simply made up of the universal elements, re-connecting with them through the practice of self-care rituals can be a humbling tool to cope with grief and loss. It can help us feel safe, trusting that it is ok to release our natural emotions to facilitate our healing.

As I watch us all aging and reflect on the ones that have left, I still recall the sounds of their voices, their laugh, echoing in my memory. I never recall any bad moments. Only the good ones. The parts of that person that brought out the joy in me. This is what humans can do for each other at their very best. Laugh, see the bright side in the darkest, saddest of times.

If there are any sensations of regret when you lose someone, think about how you can get in touch with your authentic voice. Perhaps it's time to think about how you can re-write your story about the ones you lost and the ones you still have. Did that person leave without you getting to say all the things you wanted to say to them? Were you fully expressive with them? Were you brave enough to speak your truth, as uncomfortable as it might be for you and them? If you didn't, can you see any lessons in this so that next time there is no holding you back? Are you ready to give up all the resentment or negative feeling towards them to complete your relationship with love and compassion before they pass? What if they pass unexpectedly? Did you spend your living days at peace with each other?

If we are in clear communication and undeniable honesty with those around us when we are alive, then when they are gone and we are gone, we know that we had nothing left to say to that person because we shared each other wholly and completely when it mattered most. Is it time for you to make peace with someone or something in your life? Is it time for you to let go of any fear or resentment you may have surrounding death and loss?

I AM WELLness

*'Never put the key to your happiness
in someone else's pocket'*

unknown

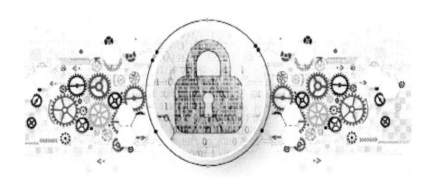

Before I developed my wellness business I had been around the houses, searching deep into my soul, falling down; bandaging my wounds; exposing them again and then healing and learning to let go of my pain and suffering. This is still in process because life carries on. Things will continue to happen; old patterns will show up and as long as we are living, we can expect the unexpected. Yet, we must still be responsible for our lives and hold ourselves accountable for our actions if we want to thrive and flourish. It has taken me years to be able to promote the many facets of wellness from the heart and from a place of truth. I have worked in environments where this word is dished out in every other sentence to try and promote something. On salon and spa treatment menus, yoga & meditation studios, and wellness retreats. It is everywhere. Online brands are now an epicentre of people (experts, and frauds alike), endorsing lifestyle and health education businesses. How do we separate the genuine from the fake? – On one hand, I have come to feel uncomfortable with the exploitation of an industry that I love so very much. The wellness market overall is a billion-dollar business and completely saturated. On the other hand, sharing this heart-centred knowledge with as many people as possible, so that we can all understand the true meaning behind 'wellness' is the goal to a global systemic shift in our awareness.

Do you remember when 'organic' became the trendy thing? Everyone, myself included, suddenly went mad for organic broccoli, eggs and milk. Then we started getting organic skincare products on the shelves in large high street pharmacy chains. We always need something new to get our consumer mind ticking.

The vegan movement came with an almighty boom to the mainstream, even though the average - Joe appears to see this as an 'extreme' lifestyle choice. That was until, we began to see the word on labels in major supermarkets. We see it on purely synthetic shower gel, knowing full well that there is nothing 'well' or natural or vegan about that product. Vegan burgers are a 'thing' that can be enjoyed not just by vegans but actual, 'old-fashioned' meat-eaters. How about it?!

In many ways, this excites me greatly. Having been a vegetarian for over 15 years, it means a lot to me that a mass consumer market becomes conscious about the detrimental effects of eating meat and questions what it means to be buying into all animal bi-products. We now have resources and access to information that we didn't have before. Search engines help to educate the consumer on how our food is being sourced and prepared. We know now that eating meat not only has major consequences for our health but also our socio-economic and environmental state. The more knowledge we have the more smoke screens we can see through and the more we shift our consciousness, getting closer to authentic living.

It wasn't until I saw the word 'wellness' advertised in a doctors' surgery that I really stopped in my tracks. What value and impact does a campaign have on the person sitting in the waiting room? 'Wellness not Illness' - a term that sums it up and seems like a very clear message. However, does this advertising campaign really help people understand the true meaning of wellness?

'Wellness not illness' as we are picking up our over the counter pharma drugs? 'Wellness not Illness' as we polish off that bottle of wine? 'Wellness not Illness' as we watch another crime drama or disturbing horror movie whilst overindulging on refined foods? And yet there is a wave of conscious living spreading across our world. Over the last two decades we have seen how people are respecting their health and seeking less mainstream approaches to having their ailments addressed, without taking the first pill the doctor prescribes. However, we are ultimately conditioned to think and act as we always have unless we are challenged otherwise. We will feed ourselves with the comforts that encourage us to feel safe and unimpeded. We will take bizarre actions to our very detriment because that is what we know. It is our comfortable junk!

I am by no means disrespecting the wonders of modern medicine, which if you break your leg; have a heart attack; need treatment for cancer; or experience a global pandemic, is there for us without question, as we see time and time again. However, what does it really take to be well and STAY WELL?

The time-honoured knowledge and practice of preventative medicine is my tool for avoiding disease, managing chronic illness and enhancing ultimate holistic health. It is sustainable and not only supports our physical problems but gives us the key to investigating our energetic body and life purpose. Win win!

Through all the peaks and troughs in my life, and through all the unravelling I have done and continue to do, I came to an understanding about myself: I had been telling myself incessantly how unwilling, unworthy and unwell I was. To be motivated enough, to be willing and worthy of my own wellness has been bumpy and disheartening. To discover that we need to actively participate in our wellness sounds like hard work and it may well be, depending on your perspective! Until, that is, it becomes a daily ritual and your lifestyle completely shifts. This only happens with repetition. Once we get into a new pattern and reiterate this on a small scale into our daily life, we then start to become what we are practicing. Rather than just dipping in and out of the latest wellness trends. When we really practice the art and science of holistic health and wellness there is a huge level of gratitude that can be accessed to re-enforce our new formed habits. Our self-belief and self-worth grow a little more every time we see and feel the difference it is making in our life.

Sometimes in this great wellness industry, our advisors and caregivers are not so connected with this idea in their own lives. Through training many therapists, I have witnessed the level of physical and mental illness within this industry and experienced it first-hand.

When you go into a spa, a clinic, or a salon, your therapist- (the one who's making you feel better, healing your pain and lightening the load) may well be approaching your energetic field with a big load of baggage of her own. If you have ever had a treatment from this person, you will know what I mean - you, the client, can feel that their heart isn't in it. You can feel that something is off, they are not concentrating or giving you a good, connected treatment.

On the other hand, your therapist may be awesome. They have so much empathy, he/she takes on all the client's pain, feels their sadness, their loss, their disease, their condition, their recent divorce. They are witness to your breakdowns, to your elation when your pain is visibly relieved after the treatment. But not every therapist is trained in counseling or practices their own self-care and therefore, the energy transfer between you both won't be synergistic, it will be one sided.

Essentially this means that you will either leave the room feeling like you wasted your money, or you will feel like you have been given a new lease of life. The therapist will either feel resentment because you have zapped all their energy and they are thinking about the six more full body massages they have to do that day, or they will be shut off and detached. It is only when there is communication and synergy between client and therapist that there can be an effective exchange which brings great healing. Both client and therapist need to take responsibility for that.

When a client comes and pays money for a service, they will gain so much more if they have a connection with their therapist rather than paying for a quick fix massage and vice versa for the therapist. I have helped people through treatment plans to recover from many different ailments. My job is to move people forward and out the other side of their perceived pain. After an initial ailment has been assessed and treated effectively there is no reason for that person to return to clinic weekly.

Maintenance is essential to keep supple, release and retune any tension or imbalance before things get out of hand but, there is a certain amount of self-responsibility that we all need to take. Our old injury or medical condition may niggle or cause chronic pain, and therefore we need to have some level of accountability for our health and wellness from all avenues. Not just nutrition from plant-based food, not only regular movement to raise the heart rate and detox. Not just manual therapy to temporarily take pain and tension away, not just meditative practice and down time, to rest. We need a small regular series of ways to constantly process the effects of life so that we can be light and feel free to re-create ourselves every time we fall down.

Wellness is a commitment and respect for our entire vessel. Wellness is being able to love and deem ourselves worthy of feeling fantastic in the many environments we are exposed to throughout our day. Wellness is knowing that we have the right to laugh and feel joy without seeking it from others as the sole pipeline and without feeling guilty or ashamed to be that for ourselves. Raising our vibration and learning self-preservation is an essential step to being independently well. Being the soul benefactor of a healthy lifestyle doesn't mean being given pills, alcohol, and negative news on a plate – all to numb our physical and mental pain and brush this precious life under the rug. Choosing REAL wellness must be driven by you. We can begin by learning one, small self-care practice at a time until it becomes part of your daily habits. Then, slowly introducing another until you have built up a holistic toolbox tailored to you. The key to living well and STAYING well is accessing something from your toolbox every day. The beauty of that is that every day, something different is available for you and will still support you on your wellness journey.

I AM accepted

'Not all those who wander are lost'
J.R.R Tolkein

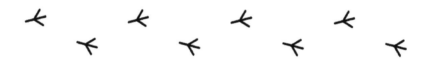

My inquiry into the deeper understanding of yogic philosophy and body therapy came around the same time as my trip to South America. I had experienced the likes of reflexology and aromatherapy treatments in previous years when I used to visit the spa with my mum. This was so helpful for my anxiety. My introduction to the power of essential oils was my access to a world where I could create and concoct. My awareness expanded as my knowledge grew. Learning phytochemistry and botany allowed me to be the scientist I never thought I was clever enough to be and the mystic witch that I always felt I was. When I got that credible pass mark in my anatomy and physiology diploma that was confirmation and proof that If I worked hard I could achieve anything. My previous experience with formal education was disappointing and now life eventually started to fall into place.

The closest I have been to experiencing pure unadulterated peace and joy was when I found my internal silence through the spiritual practice of yoga. I am not referring to yoga asanas (postures), I mean all the other facets that make up the meaning of yoga – union. After years of forcing my voice to no avail, I came to a place of not needing to be heard. I had met myself inside and paused to listen to my truth, my reality, my choices, my responsibilities and my actions; good or bad. Something I had been striving for my whole life was now unfolding. I found that 'thing' that allowed me to express myself.

Yoga was gentle and kind to me at first and then I discovered the true discipline of this spiritual philosophy. Yoga educated and liberated me. I didn't feel like a floating nomad anymore. I had the opportunity to dive deep into an ancient knowledge that has its roots in the laws of nature and the cycles of life; fundamentally encapsulating both the external and internal world we live in. I felt as though the world finally made sense in my head, heart and gut brain. Everything was connecting for me. Through intense yogic practice my body felt pain free and completely aligned. This was a miracle to me. This was my calling and having the opportunity to share this wisdom with others was a dream come true.

When I realised that people were listening for the first time in my life, I rediscovered my self-confidence that had been lost for a long time. Not the kind of confidence that entails a daily assured face that we sometimes have to force, this was a confidence I had never experienced before. One that flowed out of me, one that I trusted implicitly. This incredible spiritual awakening was enhanced by spending time in an Indian yoga ashram. However, my sense of liberty and freedom was slowly thrown out of the window as I re-entered society and had to face the reality that I left behind. I struggled to retain my deeper practice on a daily basis so I had to get creative – again and adapt my practice to suit my modern lifestyle. At first it got my back up. Reducing my yoga practice from 3-4 hours per day to only a mere 20 minutes! But, there was the test; there was the lesson, staring me in the face. I needed to show up as patient and accepting, learning to access peace in every moment at any given time, no matter the circumstance. That is the very magic of yoga.

I AM MY HEAD

*'What you resist not only
persists but will grow in size.'*

Carl Jung

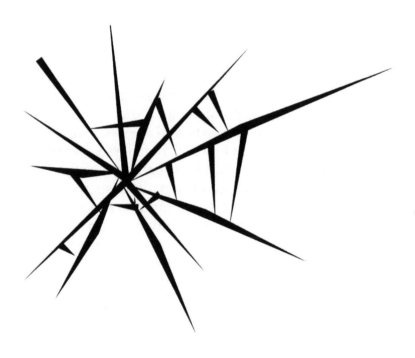

Given all of the above, my husband doesn't seem to think I am an anxious person at all! In his own words: 'I have never known anyone with the self-confidence you have'. This baffles me because nearly every moment, experience, challenge or change in my life has been riddled with some level of self-doubt, anxiety and worry. My profession is in an industry that promotes holistic health because I took a major u-turn and chose to dedicate my life to learning how to be balanced, be my best and show others the same. This very idea is riddled with questions. Is being your 'best' actually bad for you because we are striving for perfection; an ideal that doesn't exist? Maybe so. I have definitely spent time in this realm of thinking. When I say 'best' I am referring to my evolution.

I believe we are on this earth as students and I choose to never stop learning, and consequently teaching that which I have learned.

You see, fine is NEVER good enough for me anymore. I was not put on this earth to be just fine, ok or alright. I am so grateful to be here that I now don't accept anything less than fantastic! This can be exhausting though. That is another unproductive path I have been down, especially now I have two little humans to take care of. Feeling like I have to keep going and going, doing and doing, getting and getting in order to reach some kind of happiness, success or peace can be draining. How do you get to be fantastic without being exhausted all the time?

My self confidence levels have slowly risen over time but only because of immense self-reflection, analysis and growth that have put me firmly back in my rightful place. This place being my joy spark. This is my birthright. To feel joy. The place that we are all entitled to be in touch with. This re-connection with joy is sometimes not as easy as it sounds if we are riddled with mental, emotional and physical pain. If I don't practice my self-care rituals regularly, I am guaranteed to spend my days with Negative Nancy and Anxious Anne. I am never alone. I have had many days, months and years with these girls. As if life doesn't get more confusing and busier when kids come into the equation, I have these two sisters up in my face daily. What would I do without Nancy and Anne though? They really are the sisters that I never had. I have argued with them, fought them, appeased them, judged them and shamed them.

When I became a mother I realised something. I had spent my whole time searching for the next thing to achieve in life. As if I couldn't claim success until I had tangible accomplishments. College diplomas, university certificates, bigger pay checks, marriage certificates, actual real-life, self-made children who walk and talk and have their own free will. I had spent years soul searching and learning of ways to smash negativity, anxiety and self-doubt. I had spent precious time and money on training courses and traveling ventures. Looking for that 'thing' or 'one' to fill the void. Then I questioned something. Without those sisters by my side who would I be? Without my armour who would I actually be? That nice person with good intentions?

This is the part when you would normally hear that it's the doubt, fear and troubled experiences that make you the unique person you are. All the negative experiences and wounds are what makes us stronger and able to fight through. All the soul searching makes you wiser. No, no, no.

My take is this...

I have spent my life looking ahead at what I could get to be fulfilled and looking behind at what I have or haven't achieved. The sisters have been useful in my survival as a human. Being cautious and fearful has helped me avoid being run over by a bus. Being pessimistic has helped me not get let down by that new boyfriend because Nancy or Anne would pipe up and say, 'I knew that would happen' or, 'I told you so'. However, being negative and anxious has had one major impact on my life: It has stopped me from thriving and being limitless to my real human potential. And... It made me think I was singular. Special and unique in some way. A poor little victim that had all this stuff to deal with that no-one could possibly understand. I put myself in a special box and no-one had a chance of getting in.

Having children actually made me feel more of that kind of special and unique for a brief time. Although I soon realised that whilst every human is genetically and biologically unique, all I have done is add another two humans to a world of limitations and check lists. Setting them up for yet another generation of do-ers, achievers, Jones' who are all justifying their existence, doing inspirational and unique work. Supposedly special people, doing significant things.

What would happen if I finally surrendered to Negative Nancy and Anxious Anne and let go of my control freak and my go-getting, jet-setting, must-achieve-everything-to-be-accepted-in-society self? I could actually feel a sense of freedom and wholeness. I could just love them and me with all my heart. I could stop making excuses for my negative thinking or worry. I learned to do this through all-time highs and epic lows, yet loving me and them is the only way I can move forward and still feel alive and well in my life without doing a damn thing. All I needed to do is to be with them instead of fighting them and then I was released from their chains.

Have you ever contemplated what would happen to you if you were just to be? Not 'to do', but to be?

If I said, today you are going to make some white space in your diary, sit down and just be in life. What would come up for you? Would you be able to sit down in silence and feel like all is well in your world, without thinking about where you should be, what you could be doing, or what would have been done if you weren't doing this 'being' thing? Try it. Just sit down. Now, close your eyes, take a breath and just...Be...In...Life. Know that everything is well. Observe the Anxious Anne or Negative Nancy in you. What do they look like in your world? What are they telling you that you are or are not doing right? Are you going to listen to them? Or can you just ...'be'...

YOU ARE MATTER AND MIND

*'People who vibrate at the same
frequency, vibrate towards
each other. They call it, in
science, sympathetic vibration.'*

Erykah Badu

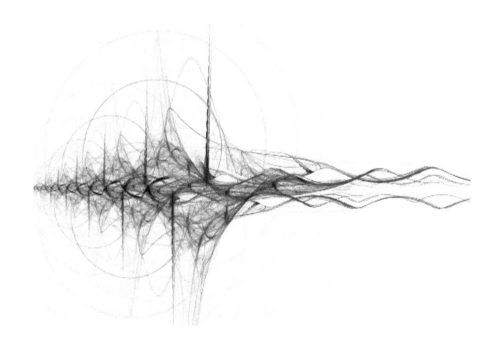

When we begin to feel aches and pains or discomfort, we are being signaled that the balance in all our intricate bodily systems is off centre. From a physiological point of view this may show in the form of overly contracted muscles or opposing slack and weak muscles. The latter can be caused by restricted posture or altered movement patterns which can happen after trauma and injury. We may be dehydrated which will affect our blood and lymph flow and reduce the amount of oxygenation in our cells and surrounding structures. We may be intoxicating our body, which again floods the body with unwanted chemicals causing fatigue, stagnation, headaches. From an energetic point of view there is less space and flow in our system. There are physical blockages which in turn may cause us to feel heavy and dense, essentially getting more and more weighed down, which will then reflect in our mental health and vice versa.

How did we get into this state? At some point (probably way back before we had that recurring back pain) we created a powerful internal dialogue to justify and govern how we are being in life. Usually this internal dialogue will be a belief we have created about ourselves and our life based on one or several negative things that happened to us. Just as I discovered when I returned to the memory of my eye surgery, and the feeling of not being heard as a child.

(Refer to chapter: I AM too little of this and too much of that, followed by my trauma memories).

When we want to communicate our worries and woes to the outside world we will simply be re-affirming that we are suffering in some way, feeding the same ongoing patterns and problems whilst continuing to ignore our bodies fundamental need to shed all the negative physical matter and low vibrational residue which would help us get back to a neutral state of being. When we start to get sick, or have stomach cramps, headaches, recurring knee, neck or shoulder pain from that 15-year-old injury, we are being reminded that this partnership between our body and mind is not being honoured and we are not taking responsibility for our health. If we are not supporting our body, we are ultimately neglecting ourselves and our potential. We often view our body as a completely separate entity to our mind.

It is even in the internal language that we speak and then re-iterate to the outside world which will be the way we live our life over and over again. Let's take the example of drinking alcohol...

'I drunk so much last night, I feel so rough. I am hungover. I vomited and can't possibly move or do anything for myself or anyone else today.'

We are talking as if it's our bodies fault and that our body has dared to fail us for having a good time last night. We laugh at our behaviours and take no responsibility for them and then we further choose to abuse our body with junk food the next day because we feel 'so bad'. Now this is not a criticism of anyone who chooses to drink and have a good time. These observations come from a lot of my own past actions and consequences.

Having been to a place of feeling systemically unwell and out of balance I am always curious as to how we talk to ourselves and how we view ourselves on that surface level.

I am going to ask you some questions for you to reflect on and answer in your own words. This exercise helps us identify with our internal dialogue and helps us see ourselves from outside of our own mind, gaining a different perspective.

1) What impact does abusive behaviour, such as binge drinking, have on your body and mind and on your vibrational energy?

....

....

....

....

2) Let's look at the actions we take. What set of low quality behaviours do you repeat over and over again, and is this conducive to a healthy mind and body?

....

....

....

....

3) Who are you surrounding yourself with? Are these people operating on a lower vibrational frequency and do you feel low after being with them?

....

....

....

....

It is important to ask why we get into our negative habits and patterns. My example of excessive drinking seems a socially common thing to do. Are we taking 'fun' to the level of destruction because we are tired, burnt out, frustrated or angry at any aspect of our life? Do we feel as if we are constantly trying to stay on top all the time, that eventually the pressure gets too much and drinking beyond what we know to be healthy, or binge eating, or using drugs is a way to release all the stored up heat and gas in our body and mind?

Do we ever have and act out the qualities of self-love and self-worth? Do we even know what that looks like? When we really ask ourselves honestly why we act the way we do is there one definitive answer or just a blurred example of moving through life, surviving, getting along, grabbing fun whilst we can, resigning ourselves to being at the effect of 'stuff' instead of homing in on our real desire to discover that 'thing' that we want and wish for in life? That 'thing' for you might feel just out of your reach and therefore forever unattainable, enough for you to settle, make do and never have the courage to go out and get what you really want.

What is that thing? Is it material wealth, successful relationships with family, friends or partners, career success, academic achievement, peace and happiness in life? Whatever it is and whatever is at the root of importance to you is personal and for you to discover. By walking through my self-care steps, identifying with the elements in the body and practicing the daily rituals, there is an opportunity for you to reconnect with your body and discover your truth.

When we make the connection that certain areas of the body correlate with one or more of the universal elements, and then apply a system of self-care designed to suit that element, we not only balance our physical selves; we also gain access to vibrant energy which allows us to fully express our aspirations and live unapologetically in our own skin.

'If only life was that easy.'

'That sounds like too much effort'

'I'm OK thank you very much'

Listening to your reactions as you read this is crucial to how you approach the next stages of the book. Do any of the above statements relate to you? What is your internal voice saying that you are then re-iterating out to the world? Whatever you are thinking is your reality. Are you completely satisfied with this? Can you see any room for growth and possibility?

Did you know that there is another way of being that doesn't involve clawing your way through the week? This 'way' is by no means easy, but it doesn't have to feel so hard. It is a choice, a discipline to direct your focus. Begin by looking at your weekly routines, habits and the language you use to describe your life. The people you choose to give your time and energy too? Are these habits serving you towards raising your vibration?

Take a good look at what you expose yourself too. Begin to establish your basic standards. Your base line. This would be the kind of information or behaviour you are willing to accept in your life and where you draw the line. Your boundaries. You can build on this standard (or reduce the filter a little, especially if it doesn't serve you in an authentic, fulfilling way). When you get focused,

Life happens. The combination of our environment, social and economic situation, family upbringing, early life experiences and influences all amount to the belief systems we have and the identity we form. This is what makes and shapes us to be the grown-up humans we are today. By being bombarded with these guidelines, we have overlooked all the other subtle factors that make us who we are. Wouldn't it be incredibly valuable for our children to be taught the knowledge of life in compulsory education? Except the last 4,000 years of history and ancient Ayurvedic wisdom isn't in our modern curriculum. We leave school knowing little about our karmic routes and our spiritual essence. We have little understanding of plant-based nutrition and how to best nourish our natural body constitution. Instead we learn the hard stuff, (literally, our physical perception of the world) the hard way first. We learn intellectual information over heart centred wisdom.

You see, the physical and material framework that we find ourselves in is our world and our reality as we think we have always known it. In western society, and from a young age, we are very quickly engineered to follow a system that has been carefully mapped out for us by our predecessors. We are taught to comply with a set of rules and conform to a range of behaviours that are deemed acceptable by the authority figures in our community. Our family lineage re-confirms that all of this is OK because we watch how the generation before us did it. Because we have emotional ties to them, we usually follow suit and don't ask too many questions. The leading figures of our family, community and religions are often the people who we look up to when we are faced with instinctive resistance or confusion about our life purpose.

Before the age of about three, human beings are somewhat exempt from all of the above. When we observe crawling babies and expressive toddlers, they are still unaware of the rule book. The world they see is full of shapes and colours which will eventually take form. The environment offers them dimension, height, textures and terrain. All of this combined with a strong will, makes for a somewhat frustrated and excitable little human. They don't yet have distinct labels for specific objects or systems, they are simply exploring their new physical world.

The yogic scriptures teach that life begins as a conscious soul travelling in the ether with no shape or form. Their karmic cycles are incomplete and so they need to return to lifeform once again. When they are conceived by life (us), they begin to take form in the womb. They had forgotten this dark place. They want to get out, so they fight their way out and accept their physical form. They arrive to this world as vulnerable physical souls who radiate light, because they are still much closer to consciousness than we are. Perhaps this is why we find babies so fascinating. They are as we often call them, 'little bundles of joy'.

Their survival is dependent on how we as their parents or carers look after them and try to impose our learned rules on them. Yet when they find their senses and their voice in the world they are still much closer to truth and joy than we are. We often say that 'children have no filter'. They have come to the earth with inherent wisdom and speak truth that we find uncomfortable sometimes. We arrived with this wisdom as well, except we have moved further and further away from our truth, hence why we experience suffering and spend the rest of our lives trying to return to it: our truth, our light and our consciousness.

I haven't met one person in my life who hasn't shared even the briefest glimmer of joy when they meet a newborn baby. People have told me that they are not maternal/paternal or they can't connect with new born babies and there is truth in this of course. They can't connect because there are too many intellectual layers in the way. I question at what stage that person is to being connected back with their own pure joy essence? As we age and go through many different life experiences, joyous and traumatic, the layers resemble our beliefs, opinions and an instinctive way of protecting our pure joy essence that we parted with when we entered the womb.

Many male clients I have spoken to have experienced a sense of detachment when being with a baby, whether it's their own or someone else's. In the rational mind, they see the contradiction from the pure bundle of joy to the painfully loud, screaming creature. It makes no sense! It isn't until the baby grows and becomes chubby, responsive, expressive and emotive that they can relate to them as a rational human being. The person that it's meant to be, in line with what we have learned.

What makes you you? Is it your parents, your siblings, your social upbringing, your religion, your routine, your education, your certificates of achievement? Your employment status, your bank balance, your material collections?

Generally, we spend our whole lives moving further and further away from our pure joy essence. When we are a child our main goal is to have fun and play. Then we are told to learn certain rules and manners which will do well for us to be accepted into our little worlds. Then we might feel resistance and unease and perhaps rebel against those rules and etiquette. We will spend most of our time comparing our beliefs, our material belongings, our opinions against others. We will find comfort in knowing that we are right and they are wrong. We will be reassured and validated by those around us that 'get it' and reinforce our 'rights' and their 'wrongs'. We become fundamentally judgmental creatures.

'How can we transform ourselves and return to joy'?

We will of course continue to watch the news, read the papers, get daily updates pinged straight to our homepage to show us all the wrongs in the world. We will find comfort in those terrible things. Reinforcing our belief that we are so lucky to live where we live and have what we have, even if yesterday we were moaning that we couldn't afford that car or house and weren't accepted for another loan or credit card. We will plod along and tell ourselves that things will get better if we just work that little bit harder and longer. This is our conditioning. Thank goodness for coffee, tea and biscuits to get us through that last shift of the week. And thank god it's the weekend. We can now relax, overindulge in a huge takeaway and consume bottles of wine because 'we deserve it'. Of course, we are fine because we had a good laugh on Saturday night. Life is good. Thank God for Sundays. We can recover, walk in a field for 45 minutes then finish off our weekend with a pub lunch and some more wine. Before we go home, make tea, eat cake and sit down in front of the tv again.

Or, Is there a small window of time when we are doing nothing? When those thoughts creep up. Those bigger questions get asked or that feeling of emptiness or curiosity creeps in? This brief window of opportunity is often a scary unknown one that we don't like the idea of facing so then boom, it's OK, our favourite show is about to come on. A perfect distraction.

'I'm tired - it's late - we've had a busy weekend and have an early start tomorrow...

Night.'
'Oh, I can't sleep. Let me pop my sleeping tablet'.

The next thing you know your alarm rings and you wonder why you feel horrendous on Monday morning?

Ah well, it's ok, we will do exactly the same thing this week and wait for a similar weekend to the last one and be grateful that we are so lucky to have this life – things could be a lot worse, so we are better off not exploring those intuitive feelings and profound questions we have about life. Yet we know that ignoring internal reflection prevents us from genuine rest, recovery, creation and innovation! But let's pat ourselves on the back for being a conditioning success anyway.

In my life before any transformation I didn't know that I had the capability to take massive action which would alter my perception of always being the victim and on the receiving end of my feelings. I did not know that if I were to take a big look at myself in the mirror, stare myself in the eyes, connect with my own deep source of power and change the language I use to describe my 'self' that this would shift my very physical and energetic vibration to one that exudes love, worth and creative expression.

Begin to recall some situations in your life that you thought would bring you a sense of happiness which, turned out to bring more stress and pressure?

....
....
....
....

List out some reasons that prevent you from 'giving up' the things or situations in your life that bring you stress and pressure?

....
....
....
....

Every cell in the body deserves nourishment and nurturing and is affected by the vibrations we expose them too. Take music and sound healing as an example. The Tibetan bowl and the gong are traditionally hand-made by the Tibetan Monks. Using a blend of raw metals from the mountains, along with hours of spiritual mantra (repeated song) it is believed to re-affirm absolute purity and healing vibrations into the instruments. When the instrument is played it gives off these high frequency vibrations which the cells in our body receive. The same applies if our body is exposed to low vibrational sound. The body will receive them, and this may have a low, negative impact on the quality of the cells. Sound baths are a great way to explore your personal experience with energetic vibration in the body.

To understand sound healing, here is an example...

Tibetan bowl playing and sound bathing with blessed instruments is the ancient equivalent to our modern ultra sound – a very popular tool used in anti-ageing skincare to help penetrate natural ingredients via sound waves deeper into the skin cells, thus giving the skin nourishment and energy. You see a visible difference in the quality of the skin after a treatment like this just like you feel an energetic difference in your whole body after a sound bath. It is truly magical because we cannot see sound yet we know its powerful effects on our cells and system as a whole.

If, through a small daily practice of self-care rituals you experienced a release in your physical and mental stress, how would you imagine that to feel like in your body, mind and life?

....

....

....

....

We must learn to be willing and ready to receive the utmost self-care into the body from a place of open heartedness and love. Being soft enough to surrender and let go of all the darkness that is stuck in the crevasses of our physical and energetic bodies. Being strong enough to stand tall and know who we are and what we are willing to give and receive from others without feeling abused or taken advantage of. We must do this with the most unconditional love for ourselves and all the souls around us if we are to discover our true joy spark again.

My interpretation of the meaning of life is to acknowledge ourselves from an authentic place of love and acceptance and then share ourselves as a gift to others. Even when they don't accept it from us. This can be the difference from a life of 'I am OK, I AM fine.' to a life of 'I AM great' and 'I AM JOY'!

When we are this way, we have raised our vibration and therefore will attract this in the universe. People will notice that you light up a room when you are this way and you will equally feel great when you light up that room!

Is there space for one thing in your life to shift? Can you write down one thing that you are willing to commit to letting go of today, that no-longer serves you and your potential greatness?

....
....
....
....

Can you write down one thing, no matter how small, that you are willing to contribute to another person today?

....
....
....
....

(When you have taken the actions on the commitments you have written down, please share this with a loved one and then record how you felt after you shared it. You can also share this with me too!

iamwellnesssolution@gmail.com

....

....

....

....

YOU ARE ENERGY

'Life, like a dome of many-coloured glass, stains the white radiance of eternity'

Percy Bysshe Shelley

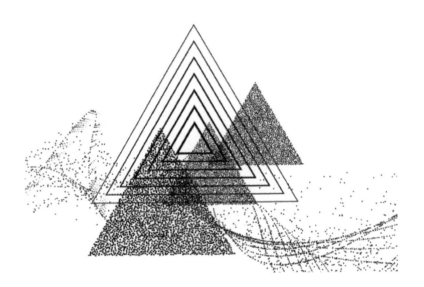

To begin this process of raising our vibration, we can start with the simple practice of smiling. This can be our symbolic baseline. Whatever is happening to you, whatever is at dis-ease in your life right now I request that you simply partake in the physical act of turning the corners of your lips up. Contracting the facial muscles is said to stimulate the system in your brain that fires up endorphins and further generates an increase in the level of happy hormones produced. Smiling is a tool I use to remind myself of what genuine peace and letting go can look like. It's sometimes necessary to use our body to trigger a certain state of being in order for us to have a start point. The physical body is a live, functioning vessel of energy which politely holds all of our negative residue in the form of toxins in our cells. We must regularly cleanse our body to bring it back to neutral so that we give ourselves half a chance to thrive clearly in the physical and mental spaces.

The five elements are located in our body and are part of the energetic chakra (wheel) system, recorded in ancient yogic scriptures over 4,000 years ago. A way to comprehend this from a modern medical perspective is by using the example of when various nerve channels, blood and lymph pathways and soft tissue junctions cross over each other creating areas of high biological and chemical activity. Of course, over 4000 years ago the yogis did not know the ways of modern science, yet somehow, without the use of microscopes and scanning devices they sourced and documented the foundations of our anatomy and physiology through their ancient visualization and deep exploration of the human vessel.

In order to understand this ancient system and how it can help re-tune our natural bodily rhythms we need to get present to the five universal elements inside and outside of our bodies.

'Earth is birth, water is growth, fire is change, air is decay and ether is death.'

The yogi understands that aside from this natural process there is an opportunity to investigate our spiritual purpose through a practical system that brings more to us than eventual pain and dis-ease which we so often resign ourselves to thinking comes with the aging process.

The system includes:

- exercise (asana)
- breathing (pranayama)
- relaxation (savasana)
- diet (sattvic)
- meditation (vedanta dhyana)

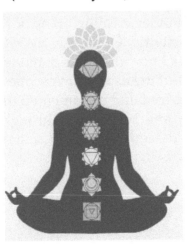

Practicing this system of simple living and high thinking gives us the access to our pathway to purity.

By becoming aware of how to work with our internal elements we will eventually, at any given time learn to help ourselves and become detached from the drama and chaos that makes us feel the weight of the world is on our shoulders. When we are having an off day where the stresses and worries of modern life are interfering with our ability to be happy and peaceful, becoming aware of the five elements and practicing gentle self-awareness helps us tune into our subtle energy – the internal state. When we remind ourselves that we do not have to be victim to, or at the receiving end of life's circumstances and the opinions of others we find transparency in some of the most threatening and challenging situations.

Gradually, with practice, we can use our energy and compassion rather than our intellect and ego to resolve and unite the challenges we experience. All whilst exuding peace and clarity. This can all be discovered by identifying with the elements and where they are located in our body. When we know their location and function, we can focus our attention on the parts of the body that need nurturing the most. We are the creators of our internal world and our external world is created by us.

I now see the chains that hook me into social conformity and material desires. Instead of being bound and oblivious to these shackles like I once was, I am now the one who holds the big ring of keys. I get to choose which chains I wish to be attached to and which ones don't serve me in any good way. I am the gatekeeper of my world and you can be too.

Let me explain what I mean when I say that I choose the chains. I got to a place in my life where I concluded that the only way I could possibly be absolutely content with my life is if I lived on a hill in the Himalayas doing four hours of yoga practice, two hours of meditation, one hour of chanting and eating only non-refined fruits and vegetables from mother nature daily. You can imagine the conundrum I faced when my Himalayan experience came to an end and I had to come back to 'reality' and society. It has taken me a long time to refine my practice and get into a self-care groove that works in my reality.

After coming face-to-face with my potential truth, or 'awakening' as some call it, the pieces of my life's puzzle slowly started coming together. There are certainly still some pieces misplaced as I navigate on my journey. Firstly, through the study of yogic philosophy, I discovered that pure bliss is not achieved by having our daily desires met. The gratification we feel when we get something shiny and new is short-lived and usually followed by a feeling of unfulfillment. This is what drives us to work towards getting something else that is shiny and new so that we can experience that sense of 'happiness' again. And so on and so forth.

Have you ever had times when you felt that something or someone really doesn't sit right with you? Quite often, we don't follow up on these instinctive feelings. We tend to hop back on that hamster wheel again. You see, unless we are sitting on that hill in the Himalayas it is very challenging to banish our egos completely from our true nature. However, we can learn the fundamentals of the ego to enable us to be eventually free from it, and still live in society, and obtain tranquility.

'Ego is the self-arrogating aspect of the mind. It separates the individual from unity with others and with the self, for the ego asserts 'I-ness'. It occupies the mind with thoughts of whether we are better or worse, possess more or less, and have greater or lesser power than others. It is attended by desire, pride, anger, delusion, greed, jealousy, lust and hatred'

– Sivananda Yoga Teachers training manual.

Our thoughts are all captives of the ego and we spend most of our lives repeating our egoic cycles until the hamster wheel gets a little bit slower, we run out of things to talk about and show off, or we just throw in the towel and give up.

The swami's / monks choose to leave their families and lives as they once knew them in a commitment to the spiritual path and overcoming the ego. They renounce all of their material attachments. This enables them to go on the pilgrimage of reaching ultimate purity which can be experienced when we transcend the senses, the intellect and ego and return to consciousness. Do you fancy going on that pilgrimage in this life? All jokes aside, this is a serious question because many people do solely choose that spiritual path.

If becoming a swami is a bit too intense yet you are intrigued and want to get closer to your spiritual essence, or, perhaps your ego has just piped up? Then, consider learning the deeper philosophy of yoga. Yoga means Union. It is the realisation of individual and universal consciousness through a direct experience. It is not the union of mind and body alone. This is a common misconception in yoga. Yoga is fundamentally spiritual.

It combines four paths of knowledge which, if in harmony, enable the individual to reach pure consciousness. And the beauty of yoga is that you can always be in practice, in any given situation.

The four main branches of yoga include –

- Karma = action: devotion to selfless service, doing duties and chores that bring you no personal gratification

- Bhakti = devotion to pure love: chanting and reciting mantra's for positive manifestation

- Raja = science: devotion to mind control by disciplining your senses and desires to banish the ego and attain clarity

- Jnana = philosophy: devotion to spiritual inquiry with continual self-examination as each new experience takes place

So, with all this knowledge we learn from the yogic scriptures, no adult can say that they are genuinely happy. It must be impossible to claim that you have attained a pure bliss state, right? We go through so much in life. It's human nature to come-up against challenges, obstacles, moments of decision, heartbreak, trauma, experiences good and bad.

Think of this as the layers being piled on top of the beautiful birth given right to be blissful. I find that so many of us spend our whole lives trying to search for that place again. That childlike playfulness and innocent joy is what we can't seem to get back to. We can't find it anymore so we either spend our whole lives searching;

filling our cup back up every time it's looking a little empty, or our whole lives compensating; ignorantly unaware of what is happening (or not happening).

It's no wonder that we jump from friendship to friendship and relationship to relationship seeking satisfaction and gratification from outside ourselves, hoping that we will fill the gap. We often do find love, we do experience moments of fun and happiness in our relationships and our friendships, we socialise, communicate and share...but for the most part this is packed in with all the other stuff that fills up life or makes us think that we are fulfilled in life. Material riches, the next holiday, the next laugh on TV. All these short-lived fixes are what makes up our lives- because we are constantly trying to re-live a sensory experience; essentially going backwards.

There is more than this. The flame of fulfillment in its true meaning is always there, whether it's small and flickering or a fearsome bonfire, it's always there. THE JOY SPARK.

The many layers I have been referring to, in yoga, are called sheaths. These are the energy fields that emit different vibrations ranging from dense (the physical body), etheric (the astral body) to vast and blissful (the causal body). Each sheath holds qualities, some of which we can relate to from a material and intuitive perspective such as the physical sheath which is made up of the five elements. The astral sheaths are made up of our breath, mind, subconscious, knowledge, ego, intellect. The most spiritual essence of us - the causal-sheath can be accessed by committing to lifelong introspective practice with the mission to arrive at a level of consciousness beyond what our rational brain alone can comprehend. (The thing the swamis and monks do). This takes immense discipline and renunciation, with the goal of enlightenment and release from this physical world entirely. (Never to return inside the karmic cycle again). Anyone can make the choice to follow this spiritual path, yet it sounds intense and scary.

For now, we will begin to understand the basic concept of the five elements and five senses.

Discovering how to tune into this elemental level will enable you to form a baseline in which to manage the dissatisfactions and frustrations you face, move through any blockages or mindsets that are holding you back and fulfill on your individual goals and self-development. With practice, there will be a slow shift in your gross body, in your energy body and you will get a deeper sense of purpose whilst being fully present in your world and without having to disappear into the mountains for the rest of your life – unless you choose the ultimate spiritual path of course! You can be spiritually awake as well as functioning and flourishing in your material world, starting with being kind to ourselves.

YOU ARE A GIFT TO YOURSELF

'The intuitive mind is a sacred gift. The rational mind is a faithful servant. We have created a society that honours the servant and has forgotten the gift.'

Albert Einstein

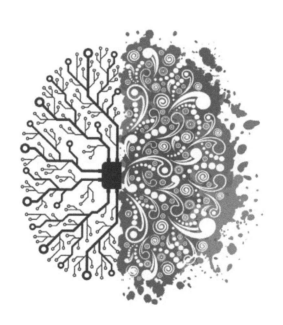

When we learn about the elements within the chakra system we begin from the ground up…

EARTH

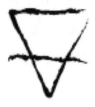

Chakra/ Location in body – Coccygeal/sacral plexus/ buttocks & legs

Relationship/Association to the physical world – All solid material discovered in the solar system: from the rocks that make up the planets to the coral in the seabed; mother of pearl, to the bricks that build our houses.

Sense - Smell

Organ/gland - Adrenal glands, colon, spine, perineum

Balanced - Safe and stable

Imbalanced - Indecisive, low mood

Qualities – Being strong and supportive. Making a stand for your values and principles. Providing crucial life force in the way of stem cells to the entire defence (immune) system in your body.

When we are aligned with our earth centre we have a strong connection to our roots. Our basic human needs are being met and there is a sense of ritual and discipline in our life.

The earth centre can be disturbed when we travel or move around a lot. Changing jobs, locations and relationships can all play a part in unsettling the earth centre.

Exercise:

Sitting still, in a safe space, begin to quieten the internal dialogue for a moment. Imagine your physical entity and your busy mind sitting together: A solid container which holds the five key components that make up 'YOU'.

Bring your attention to your feet and your bottom, sitting on a seat or touching the ground. As if you have x-ray vision, look inside the physical body for your bones. All parts of you that are made up of a bony/cartilage material, from the tiny bones in your feet up to the largest bones in your legs. Ask yourself - do my bones care that I didn't get that promotion? Or, do my bones get upset that my kids didn't listen to me this morning? No, our bones don't have those feelings.

Our whole body subtly responds to all vibrations that pass through it - high and low feelings. Sadness, chronic stress, abusive language will give off an energetic vibration which will distribute all the way into the cells that make up your bones. Just as joy, laughter and high vibrational language will do the same and with a greater effect on your wellbeing. We need to acknowledge the basic qualities of the bones and honour them kindly.

The bones are our earth. Like all food that's made up of naturally occurring material will decompose into the earth and becomes the earth - so do our bones. Our bones are the physical matter that become the ground that we walk on. Sitting still on the ground is a great way of connecting to our earth and our micro/macro connection.

At times of fear and change when we are thrown off course, we may experience being more scared, stressed and unstable in life.

Ask yourself - do you trust the ground you walk on or do you feel shaky and unsafe?

How to stay stable when things are out of your control-

Have you ever experienced upheaval in your life? Have you noticed that whatever the initial upheaval was- it has been the subtle blueprint to how you react to subsequent upheavals?

When we are safe, stable and comfortable, our guard is down and we are usually relaxed and open minded. We are rooted and can be productive and pragmatic. When we are faced with a threat, our natural instincts react with our primitive fight, flight or freeze response. This could be translated to being on the attack, on the defense or paralysed in a non-communicative, state. The fight, flight and freeze state is fundamental for our inherent need to survive, yet it is not usually relevant to the everyday stresses we may experience in life or at all helpful for our growth. For example – A situation in the office nowadays might make us react similarly to how our ancestor would have when she was faced with an attack from wolves in her camp. The more stress we incur in modern life, the more our primitive functions will heighten.

Our first energy centre in our body is home to our adrenal glands, spine, large colon and bones. It is imperative that we restore our earth energy in order to grow. Just like a blossoming flower starts as a seed in the earth, we need to visualize this space in our physical body as our anchor. When we connect to the idea that we are anchored, how does that leave us? Secure, strong and stable. Even the sound of the word 'anchor' has an unbreakable tone to it. When we don't relate to this space consider that we are going through life with a weak backbone. There may be a lack of self-worth and integrity. When we restore our roots, and re-discover where we came from, we instill discipline into our lives and our basic human needs can be met in order for us to rise.

Now consider that in our life from a young age, our roots are guaranteed to be disturbed by something and we will experience fear or insecurity in some capacity. If this isn't addressed it can manifest persistent low mood, indecisiveness and lead to deeper conditions such as depression and mood disorders.

Can you relate to this in your life? Do you see yourself as someone with a strong anchor who is rooted, yet free to move and change without being debilitated by fear? When we begin to relate to the elements concept in our physical body (the earth being the first) we can connect to our source of stability and strength in life from the ground upwards. When we are in balance this we can build on it, gradually traveling up through each element, getting clarity and balance within each space until we reach a state of physical and mental harmony.

Do you want to be decisive and confident in your life?

Refer to chapter – 'YOU ARE a ritual'
Your core practice = The five EARTH exercises in steps 1-5.

WATER

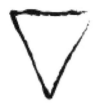

Chakra / Location in body – Sacral / lumbar / hypogastric / renal plexus & lower back

Relationship/Association to the physical world – All fluid material in our solar system. From the smallest droplet of morning dew found on a blade of grass, to our mighty rivers and oceans, to the running water that comes from our taps.

Sense - Taste

Organ/gland - Reproductive system, bladder & kidney

Balanced - Creativity and joy

Imbalanced - Fearful and bogged down

Quality - Flowing through life with ease. Letting go of toxicity and trusting the process. Being confident in our creativity. Experiencing joy and purity. Smooth delivery of physical nourishment to our cells via the circulatory system and lymphatic system whilst collecting waste product that our body (and mind) no longer need by filtering and eliminating.

Have you ever been in an experience where you feel free and able to let yourself go? This is very different from being irresponsible and reckless, although the two often get confused.

When we are aligned with our water centre, we feel like we flow through life with ease. Our creativity thrives and there is an authentic sense of joy within us.

The water centre can be disturbed when we experience emotional trauma, abuse or addictive tendencies. Inevitably our 'taste' and 'desires' for life get triggered into over-drive or under-drive here. If you are thrust into a situation that is out of your control or have heavy responsibility and duties to attend to this can bear a significant burden on the creative centre.

This area of the body and energy will be thrown out of balance leaving us feeling bogged down, fearful and innovatively stunted.

When we let our inhibitions go, we may feel that we will get betrayed or hurt again. Have you ever experienced this? Have you ever been in a situation and felt that you can't let go fully because you don't want to expose yourself or show vulnerability?

To have unlimited resources of joy, time and time again, after judgments, trauma and let down, you must ultimately learn to let go of whatever it is you are holding so tightly to. Whether this relates to someone not meeting your expectations or something in your life that is unfinished business. As terrifying as it is, you must face it and ask yourself this – Am I brave enough to let go? If I let go, what will happen to me? Can I forgive?

Are you going to die on the spot if you let go of this stress? Is this trauma or unfinished business even relevant to your life anymore? If not, why are you bringing it into your present life? It is stunting your creativity and self-expression. If the 'thing' you are not letting go of is still relevant, then what pro-active plan do you have in place to prepare to let it go in the future? What help and support do you need? The reason I say 'thing' is because this will be a different event, situation or person for everyone. It is usually the bugbear that is always showing up in your inner dialogue. It is usually the reason for your biggest fears in life. Try exploring what your 'thing' is. As we touched upon in the chapter: YOU ARE the Joy Spark.

Remind yourself, what you are willing to forgive and let go of? What would it feel like to be free from your shackles?

Being terrified and controlling blocks your creative flow and will cause a chronic backlog in your life and in the relevant area of the body. Eventually the beautiful river of joy that you are, intrinsically, will become a smelly, stagnant, bitter pond of resentment and the same goes for your fluid system. Our physical body is made up of 70% water. When our lymphatic system is slow and sluggish, it is unable to clean out our system effectively, resulting in toxic residue and illness. Imagine all the juices in our container begin to smell and seep toxicity into all other organs, glands and spaces in the body. This is not a river I would like to swim in!

We see how children are beautiful, creative creatures. They are fully flowing through life with so much to explore and express. Yet, more often than not, we somehow think it's our right to channel and divert them, even stop them in their tracks and send them on a path that arguably was never designed for them. The 'right' path. The 'socially acceptable' path governed by duty and order. I question this path because in my own experience this wasn't suited to my nature. I know that my anxiety began when I felt I was failing in life and not meeting expectations or achieving as I perceived everyone else to be. Our children must find their own path and be set free. Yet, we must be right there, by their side and ready to support them when they have their falls.

Do you want to move through life freely and with creative abundance?

Refer to chapter – 'YOU ARE a ritual'

Your core practice = The five WATER exercises in steps 1 -5.

FIRE

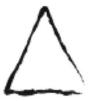

Chakra / Location in body –Solar / celiac plexus / middle thoracic & abdomen

Relationship/Association to the physical world – All hot material: from the blazing fires in every star, to our sun; the bubbling magma in the earth's crust, to the candle we burn on our kitchen table at night.

Sense - Sight

Organ/gland - Pancreas, liver, intestines, stomach

Balanced - Strong and active

Imbalanced - Fatigued, dis-empowered

Quality – The internal torch that gives you energy through digestion and metabolism. The fire in your belly. A forever flickering flame of potential power within you. On your darkest days the flame will be dim and until your physical matter passes from this world, never put out.

When we are aligned with our fire centre we feel as though we can accomplish anything. We are leaders and take big action to achieve our goals. We have vibrant and crucial energy.

The fire centre can be disturbed when we get humiliated or our pride is shattered, leaving us powerless and lethargic.

In the physical – we nurture our fire centre with quality nutrition that comes from whole foods which exude a high vibration of energy. It is alive. If we regularly eat food that is processed, refined and mainly made of sugar or salt- essentially low vibrational, we are depriving our gut from functioning optimally. This whole fire system will become depleted and reliant on quick fixes.

In order to get real with our health we need to take an honest look at our life. This centre also governs the sense of sight so if we are fatigued here, we may also be blindsided or have a distorted view of how the world sees us. If we cleanse our gut, flush our body with nourishing foods, we will gain clarity and energy to become a powerful and productive leader.

What will you do with your power?

Have you ever come across that confident person who we all know is actually cocky and arrogant? An example of when your third energy centre is out of balance is when your power becomes too hot and toxic. This type of power likes to dominate and control situations.

It is possible to feel completely empowered with good, abundant energy. It is possible to be assertive without being aggressive. It is possible to see a situation for how

it really is rather than through rose tinted glasses...
Regardless of any criticism you may receive.

Do you want to ignite the fire back into your belly and channel your power?

Refer to chapter – 'YOU ARE a ritual'

Your core practice = The five FIRE exercises in steps 1-5.

AIR

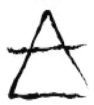

Chakra / Location in body – Cardiac / pulmonary / brachial plexus / upper thoracic & arms

Relationship/Association to the physical world – The finest material in the solar system. From the poisonous gases released from the sun to the soft clouds above us, to the oxygen we breathe into our lungs.

Sense – Touch

Organ/gland - Heart, thymus, lungs

Balanced - Compassionate, empathetic

Imbalanced - Resentful & jealous

Quality – These most subtle life-giving molecules are selflessly floating around, waiting to be inhaled and exhaled. This is the giving and receiving nature of the heart and lungs which is parallel to the simple transaction of energy that all living organisms partake in order to stay alive.

When we are aligned with our air centre, we are breathing freely without restriction. Much like our lungs and surrounding muscles expand and contract, so does our heart energy.

The air centre can be disturbed when we experience loss, grief and heart break. This place in our body is symbolic of the duality of life. This begins simply by knowing that all things begin as masculine and feminine. The sun and moon are examples of the natural sources of masculine and feminine energy. The sun is hot and aggressive. When we look at the nature of our masculine organs in the body we see that the gall bladder, stomach, intestines and bladder generate heat. The moon is cool, and passive by nature. The organs and glands in the body that are feminine are the kidneys, the heart, liver, lungs and spleen: The inhale and exhale; Yin and Yang; Ida and Pingala; up and down. The polarity theories may have different terminology or may be written in a different language, yet they all have something in common: They all resonate towards masculine and feminine energy within nature. All equating to the same meaning.

Our emotions are the same. We sway from angry to melancholy. From happy to sad. When we experience grief in our life our heart energy is pulled up and down and left and right and our emotions can overwhelm us. When there is disharmony or disease our heart energy is the central vortex in our body where upward and downward flowing energy meet. There can be huge clashes here. Jealousy, anger and toxicity can develop if we don't deal with our neglected hearts.

The answer is forgiveness. Forgiveness and acceptance is the only way we can come back to harmony with our heart centre.

If we ignore or abuse the air element and it's associations, we forget the sacredness of our breath; the life giving force that we cannot live without.

Do you want to be compassionate and abundant in love?

Refer to chapter – 'YOU ARE a ritual'

Your core practice = The five AIR exercises in steps 1-5.

SPACE

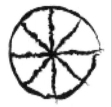

Chakra / Location in body – Pharyngeal / cervical plexus / throat & neck

Relationship/Association to the physical world – Space, the atmosphere, the sky, the ether that fills everything in between all solid matter in the world and is the bridge to our spiritual essence that we cannot see with the naked eye.

Sense - Hearing /Sound

Organ/gland - Thyroid, parathyroid, auditory system

Balanced - Optimum capacity to listen and communicate honestly

Imbalanced - Over talking/over thinking/ frustrated

Qualities – This space is our path to self-expression and our portal to the third eye and crown chakra that cannot be accessed wholly without deep meditation, stillness and balance throughout the first five elementary systems.

The space centre can be disturbed when we have too much cerebral chatter in our mind. We often judge people's abilities by their intellectual capacity. Certain tests and studies carried out by psychologists can vouch for levels of intelligence but often fall short and don't cover the wide range of human skill sets, from both creative/subjective and intellectual/objective perspectives. We know that these 'clever tests' were designed by pre and post WW2 white, middle aged men and usually for the purpose of the armed forces. These narrow and limited assessments are now outdated and biased.

The dominant subjective mind is often emotionally intuitive. The dominant objective mind is information-intelligent. One is not better than the other. We need a balance and when the mind gets overcrowded, with either too much fantasy or too much fact, there will be a disparity in the space element and corresponding organs and glands. When we are aligned with our space centre our knowledge is working simultaneously with our actions and we can start to live without judgement of others. We can be our word. We can practice what we preach. With true conviction.

Once we begin to regularly practice attuning ourselves to the five elements and the five senses inside our body, we start to see the unparalleled synergy that exists within our human form and in our universe.

We develop a knowledge that there is more to the human capsule than all our junk, our blame, our reasoning, our mind, our intellect and ego that we carry so heavily around with us.

When we become aligned to our internal microcosm, it is possible to gain a wide perspective on every tiny detail in our life alongside every huge one. From this new standpoint it is now conceivable that there is another space in our body, our mind, our hearts, where real peace and fulfillment lives. This space is sacred to you and only you. No amount of external influence or invasion can enter your space unless you let it. Even when your senses, your emotions, all of your human reactions try to defend or attack the outsider, the 'you' that is found in your sacred space is unattached and completely at ease. This is 'You' transformed.

Do you want to reveal your true self and express with ease in life?

Refer to chapter – 'YOU ARE a ritual'

Your core practice = The five SPACE exercises in steps 1-5.

As we now move into the five core holistic health rituals, it is vital that whilst we retain the new information, we keep returning to our sacred space, in order to allow room for all the transformation to take place!

YOU ARE a ritual

'Rather than criticizing others, we should evaluate and criticize ourselves. Ask yourself, what am I doing about my anger, my attachment, my pride, my jealousy? These are the things we should check in our day to day lives.'

Dalai Lama

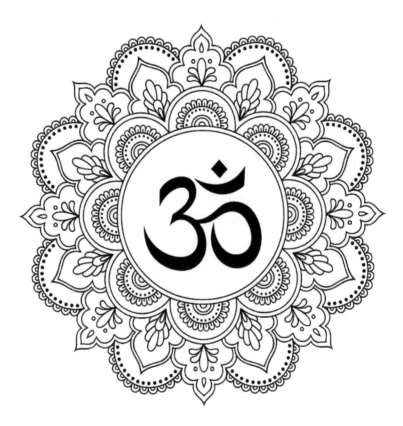

The Rituals

1) Affirmation - A willingness to express with conviction and in words, that which you want to attain.

2) Self-Massage - A productive approach to get hands-on in all areas of the elemental body.

3) Yogic exercise - A connection with the breath in order to stay in a flowing, pain reduced state.

4) Sattvic nutrition - A commitment to nourishing and fueling your body with pure foods.

5) Self-care - A willingness to cleanse your head, heart and gut through loving your skin.

STEP 1 - Affirm

You are being your word

When we are feeling worried or sad, grieving or going through a personal trauma and someone tells us to 'stay positive' this can do more harm than good. The 'stay positive' response feels extremely cliché to me these days. Opening up to the idea that thinking positively helps us overcome some of life's obstacles certainly serves a purpose. Yet, to understand how to stay positive we need to actually be positive. To understand how to be positive is to start listening, to start listening requires action and taking responsibility! Actively listening to our own internal dialogue is a crucial way to decipher what is really holding us back and keeping us in a negative loop.

The other concept we need to grasp is learning how to tune into others. Listening to others is really hard. We humans are great at hearing (assuming our auditory system is functioning well) yet generally terrible at really listening. Do you know why? Because our internal dialogue is so loud, we are too busy responding to that instead. What does she think of me? Do I look fat in this outfit? Did I say something stupid? I did this, I did that, I am going here and I am going there… I can't even remember what she was talking about.

We need to ask ourselves when was the last time we gently connected with someone with eye to eye contact, kept our mouth shut and let them say what they had to say for longer than 30 seconds with genuine compassion? When there was a natural pause in the conversation did we pursue what they were talking about for them or, did we think of something relevant to say about ourselves and start talking about that instead? It's at that point that the conversation turns. We have potentially killed off any real communication with that person. We need to explore this listening game! Once we get good at this there will be a huge difference in the way we attend to ourselves and attend to others in our life.

Since most of us don't have the time, patience or inclination to go into a deep meditative practice or embark on a spiritual journey into the listening of others, I will just say this....

The quickest and easiest way to 'stay positive' and adjust our outlook when it comes to obstacles, people and situations that life throws at us is to find something to say that is in-line with our truth and then practice saying it out loud.

Affirm it! This is very different from gossip, small talk, showing off or the other extreme of playing yourself down to others. You might even find this to be incredibly confronting. I cannot express the importance of this practice enough, though. This is where real personal power is. Expressing your truth to yourself first and then to your world.

By the time you have got this down you will find that the conversations you have with others shift. They no longer revolve around your worries, your woes and all your venting. You actually become attuned to listening to others and holding a clear space for them whilst preserving your sacred space. You may even find that having nothing to say for yourself on a topic of conversation is more productive and peaceful than saying something just for the sake of it. You may even want to share this practice with them at a later time. The other person may then discover something new about you to help them understand and hear themselves clearer than ever before.

It all starts with **affirming to self.**

The practice of affirmations is an ancient ritual for many cultures. A 'mantra' is a statement or word in the form of sound, repeated frequently to aid concentration on an intention that the person chanting the mantra wants to manifest. This suggests there is an element of focus and discipline needed when you start your affirmation journey.

When we feel stressed out with a work project or colleague, the kids are doing your head in or you have something niggling away at you like 'should we move house, should I look for another job, should I have that conversation with that friend' we tend to fall into a habitual way of thinking about how to solve these problems. We might get highly emotive, letting our feelings take over and talk for us, or we might get a case of what I call 'the super cerebral' when your intellectual mind is the dominant conversation in your head. How can Mrs Super Cerebral resolve this problem pragmatically, rationally and logically we ask ourselves, whilst bashing Mrs Super Cerebral's very smart head against a solid brick wall!

Let's not get interested in any of that noise now. Let's instead cast all that exhausting chatter aside. Let's just get real and get true. What is bothering you and what do you really need to do to achieve your goals and move forward towards what you want in life?

Ask yourself right now and note it down.

What is it at the forefront of my mind that is bothering me?

....

....

....

....

Case studies

Client - Lucy (30 years old, mum of two) –

'I am so tired. My toddler has not slept through the night since she was born. I spend my nights settling her several times and then getting up to go to the loo, then my brain is alert so I can't get back to sleep and then before I know it I am getting up with my 4 year old at 6am as he has always been an early riser. I never actually feel like I sleep. I find it hard to relax in the day because I need to do the washing, prepare the dinner, clean the house, feed the baby, collect my child from school.'

Lucy's internal mantra is - I am so tired. I am so tired. I am so tired. I can't relax. I can't relax. I can't relax.

Affirmation exercise for:

Re-grounding

Whenever Lucy feels the urge to express how tired she is to her husband, her mother, her sister, her friend and even herself I asked her to do the following....

'Lucy, find a private space and stand still. Place both hands behind your back and into the lowest part of your spine. (the earth / root centre) Be silent for a few seconds and repeat to yourself internally three times...

'STOP, STOP, STOP'.

Now, if you feel comfortable close your eyes. Take a deep breath in and then as you breathe out repeat...

'I am grounded, I am grounded, I am grounded.' Repeat two more rounds of this.

You see, Lucy never stops. Lucy is officially 'on one'. She is frustrated. She is overwhelmed and, you guessed it, horrifically tired. Lucy knows all of this but is struggling to be heard and there doesn't appear to be a solution to her problems. So, she is on a habitual loop. 'I AM tired. I AM tired. I AM tired.' Everything feels unfair to her.

Unless Lucy wants to be on this loop, or a variation of this loop for the rest of her life the only thing she must do now is actively change the record.

Since Lucy began introducing these small daily rituals, she is learning to speak differently about her state of energy. Although the physical sensations of tiredness are there, she is choosing to speak words that enhance her energy levels such as –

'I am breathing in energy' rather than repeatedly reinforcing her suffering by speaking those debilitating words 'I am tired' to no productive avail!

Client – Stephanie (45 years old, working professional)

'I have been so busy at work lately plus going to loads of events in the evenings. I do my class on Thursdays which I love, it is my escape, unlike being at home. My husband just doesn't seem to get me lately, or care that much. He's so boring and stuck in his routine. It feels like we are growing apart'.

Stephanie's internal mantra is - 'I am unnoticed. I am unloved. I am too busy'. In fact, so busy that there does not seem to be any time or room to accept any love.

Affirmation exercise for:

Forgiving

Every time Stephanie accepts to work late, go to that event, or do her class, she deprives herself of consciously being with her husband. Stephanie is also stuck in her routine and equally not paying attention to her husband. I asked her to do the following...

'Stephanie, find a private space and stand still. Place both hands in the centre of your chest (air / heart centre). Be silent for a few seconds and repeat to yourself internally three times...

'FORGIVE. FORGIVE. FORGIVE.'

Now, if you feel comfortable close your eyes. Take a deep breath in and then as you breathe out repeat...

'I am open, I am open, I am open.' Repeat two more rounds of this.

We discovered that Stephanie just wants to feel loved and appreciated. She is always so preoccupied saying 'yes' to everything that she feels overused and struggles to set boundaries. Stephanie is actually hard on herself and then goes home and doesn't get the attention or reaction that she expects from her husband. This reinforces their disconnect and they continue to be in a habitual loop of avoiding communication.

The moment she begins to open up authentically with her husband about her needs, there will be a new powerful space created for her relationships and priorities to really shift.

Exercise –

Choose a core affirmation from below.

In a moment, close your eyes. Take a deep inhale. Take a deep exhale. Repeat your chosen one three times, taking a full inhale and exhale after each repetition.

Gradually introduce a second, third, fourth and fifth affirmation into your daily rituals. From earth to space, begin to 'say your way' to complete elemental balance.

Earth - Ground yourself - 'I AM GROUNDED'

Water - Find your fluidity - 'I AM FLOW'

Fire - Digest and perform - 'I AM ENERGY'

Air - Be forgiving - 'I AM OPEN'

Space - Discover your self-expression- I AM TRUTH'

Step 2 – Self massage

You are connecting with the vessel

Massage has been a primary self-care practice dating back to the Egyptians and ancient swamis. When massage becomes part of our regular lifestyle habits, we start to see it as practicing an art form. Building regular massage practice into your life is a profound creative process in discovering your body. Whether it's a therapist giving you a beautifully connected treatment, or learning how to self-massage, this must be celebrated as a sacred act of self-love. When we pay attention to our well-being needs, we have the ability to maintain and manage our own aches, pains or old injuries. This is a chance for us to be fully engaged in the nursing of ourselves physically and metaphysically through the form of touch therapy.

To balance our internal elements through massage requires an understanding of how the different parts of our body relate to the distinct characteristics of each of our energy centres.

Earth – physical stagnation and lethargy -

Massage location - Legs and feet

Area of energetic rebalance - Pharyngeal / cervical plexus

When I work with clients who suffer with depression and low mood some common symptoms I see in the body are dehydrated soft tissue and an imbalance in oil production in the skin. Often a combination of dry and oily in various locations.

If there is instability in the base/earth centre, feelings of being heavy and stuck, there will likely be instability in the mind. Starting with the feet and legs, I almost always encourage blood and lymph flow to the area with a gradual upward movement throughout the whole body, towards the groin, abdomen and neck where there are major lymphatic drainage sites. This is a valuable way to revive the mood and bring clear energy to the entire system.

Exercise – home massage technique –

- You can regularly connect with the feet by sitting in a lotus position or getting as comfortable as possible in a seated position on the floor with your legs in front of you. Ideally with a wall behind you to support your back from hunching over.
- Take one foot at a time, resting it onto your opposite thigh and firmly hold it with both hands for a few seconds. This is a great way of initially checking in with your mental state. Breathe in and out here.
- You can then apply your chosen body oil or scrub over the whole foot and lower leg (one foot at a time) making sure you thoroughly rub the toes, heels, and ankles. Continue this for up to 10 minutes.

(Note – stop the massage techniques if you feel any pain)

Water – subconscious suffering and unaddressed trauma

Massage location - groin, buttocks, lower back

Area of energetic re-balance – Solar / celiac plexus

The sacral area is a sensitive and somewhat vulnerable place in the body. For men and women, it is the centre of the reproductive organs, creativity, the source of life-giving energy. If my client has had trauma in the form of deprivation or addiction, giving body work to this area can metaphysically open up Pandora's Box. This can be a gentle and nourishing experience to help release restriction affecting the surrounding structures and soft tissue. Energetically though, the client may be left with a sense of crisis as dormant energies begin to open up and old memories are revived.

When massaging the sacral area, I advise a course of treatment where there is continued attention focused on the lower back, moving into the middle back. From a face-up (supine) position the attention is focused in the hip flexors, lower abdomen then up into the solar plexus and ribs. Any subconscious energy released from here needs to go somewhere. Channeling it into the solar plexus can help the client process and manage any old trauma that may be released. This may help encourage them to see and communicate their needs when they feel ready to do so. I have referred clients to colleagues who specialise in mental health therapy and always encourage the two modalities to work alongside each other for additional support. Often, what can't be expressed in words, is revealed through integrated body therapy.

Exercise - home massage technique –

- Begin by getting into an upright kneeling position. (Use a mat or cushion under the knees for support) Before you massage this area it is important to check in with your posture. Gently tuck the tailbone in, engage the stomach muscles and roll the shoulders back. With both hands in a clenched fist position, slowly and softly pummel/tap the lower back and glutes with an alternating movement.
- When you get into a comfortable rhythm you can gradually increase the pressure and speed of the pummeling/tapping. This can also be done over your lower abdomen and the front of your thighs and hips.

(Note – stop the massage technique if you feel any pain)

Fire – Anger and irritation

Massage location - stomach, middle back

Area of energetic re-balance – Cardiac /pulmonary / brachial plexus

If I am presented with a client who is pre-disposed to inflammatory disease, reactive to heat or has allergies, my first assessment would be on their gut and their diet. Ayurvedic diet analysis helps determine if the foods we eat are complementary or counterproductive to our natural body constitution. If there is suffering in this area of the body, it can often be associated with mood swings, skin flare ups and stomach conditions such as I.B.S, heartburn and auto-immune disease. Initial massage around the stomach and middle back will be hugely beneficial to support and relieve the physical conditions that come with the latter ailments. However, the area of energetic re-balance usually lies within the cardiac plexus. The heart centre. Massaging through the stomach and then up and around the chest and lungs gives our nervous system a chance to stabilise.

To support any inflammation means bringing the body into an alkaline state through parasympathetic nervous system (rest and digest) encouragement and efficient diet. In other words, lowering acidity and cooling the heat produced when the sympathetic nervous system is in overdrive (fight/flight/freeze). Balancing the heart energy is a wonderful healing support for inflamed bodies and aggravated minds.

Exercise - home massage technique –

- The stomach massage is most effective when you are lying down on your back in a resting state. Either first thing in the morning or last thing at night. Make sure your legs are apart and bring both hands to the centre of your stomach, resting under your ribcage. Take a breath here.

- Slowly move both hands to the left side of your stomach and press gently and repeatedly in the space between the hip bone and ribs. The more familiar you get with your body the deeper you can press. This will stimulate your large intestines and help any trapped air move through the colon. Bring the hands back to the central stomach area, resting them under your ribcage. Now, repeat the massage on the right side, in the space between the hip bone and ribs. This will stimulate your stomach, liver and small intestines – encouraging undigested food to move through the gut with more ease.

(Note – stop the massage technique if you feel any pain)

Air – Emotional upheaval -

Massage location - rib cage, upper chest and upper back

Area of energetic re-balance - Coccygeal / sacral / lumbar plexus

For someone who is emotionally unbalanced, experiencing hormonal changes, grieving or has physical ailments such as asthma or lung conditions I would work with soft tissue techniques around the rib cage, upper chest and upper back/shoulders in order to ease physical tightness, wheezing and mucous build up. Then the focus may needs to be brought to the buttocks, lower back and hip flexors – the area that often causes our upper posture to become weak and depleted or alternatively hypertonic due to repetitive strain habits and psychological inattention.

Nourishing the heart centre is also one of the most comforting ways to support someone who has experienced emotional pain and loss. It can initially feel sensitive to receive treatment to this area because the air element directly relates to the sense of touch. Yet, the burdens that get lifted after a few sessions of paying tactile attention to the heart, is incredibly healing.

Exercise - home massage technique –

- Place both hands on the centre of the chest for a moment whilst you find a slow, calm breathing pattern. With one hand on top of the other, gently press your flat palms into the chest, gradually applying more pressure. Release after 5 seconds. Move both your hands to the right side of the chest (on top of the pectoralis muscle) and repeat the technique. Move both your hands to the left side of the chest and repeat this technique.

(Note – stop the massage technique if you feel any pain)

Space – Mental distress or fatigue

Massage location - shoulders, neck, throat and head

Area of energetic rebalance - Coccygeal/sacral plexus

When someone has signs of high-functioning anxiety and unease, root grounding the legs and feet helps to stabilize the nervous system, drawing energy away from the head and towards the base. Generally, the shoulders, neck, throat and head accrue physical tension when we experience acute stress and anxiety which, if not addressed, will manifest into chronic stress and other health conditions.

Giving traditional soft tissue massage to this area is extremely beneficial. However, considering a more subtle approach such as cranio-sacral therapy can be the difference between simple pain maintenance and genuine nervous system healing. Cranio-sacral therapy helps relieve pressure in the sinuses and the sutures of the cranium and sacrum. This type of therapy also works on a subtle level, moving and shifting fluid deep within the spinal cord and in turn, releasing physical and mental limitations.

Exercise - home massage technique –

- Cranio-sacral therapy must be carried out by trained professionals. However, certain pressure point can be located in the shoulders and neck and combined with gentle massage are a great way to relieve physical tension.
- Bring your left hand to the left shoulder and your right hand to the right shoulder. Bring your fingers together and press them firmly into the large shoulder muscle (trapezius) several times. You may find lots of tightness and tension in this area. Gradually walk your fingers up to either side of the neck and firmly press the fingers along the neck (either side of the spine). Move your fingers further up the neck until you reach the base of the skull. Repeatedly press and rub into where the head and neck join.

(Note – stop the massage technique if you feel any pain)

Step 3 – Movement and breath

You are disciplining and regulating the internal systems

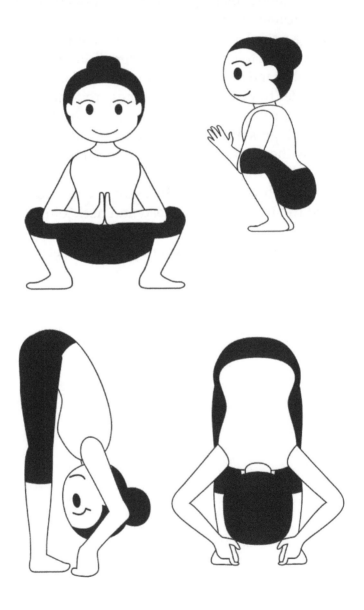

All yoga asana's (postures) and pranayama's (breathing exercises) are designed to support specific areas in the body, mind and energy system. That is why yoga is a truly holistic practice. We are not just sweating and releasing endorphins when we practice yoga. We are purposefully exploring the subtle internal world and supporting our entire system to work in synergy.

Earth exercise – Standing forward bend/big toes pose (uttanasana /pada hastasana) and prayer squat (malasana)

- Start by simply squeezing the tummy muscles, bend the knees and roll the body forward into a folded, hanging rag doll. Drop the head and arms towards the ground and gently move your back from side to side to feel a nice stretch. Keep the feet firmly planted on the ground.
- Come back to the centre bending position and tuck the chin to chest. Take a deep inhale and exhale and hook your index and second finger under the big toes on both sides. Keep the knees bent if the stretch is too restricted at first. Gradually begin to straighten the legs as your practice evolves.

This is a great warm-up exercise before starting any yoga asana practice. This grounding technique aims for us to reach for the earth, stretching out the spine from the top of the neck to the bottom of the coccyx.

- Continuing, gently open the feet wider. Bend into the prayer squat and place your hands on the floor to support your balance. Always breathe slowly in and out during the sequence.
- When you are steady in your squat, slowly bring your hands to prayer position on your chest.

- Over time, encourage your arms to move inside of the thighs, prayer hands pushing against each other, as you lift up your chest, roll the shoulders and straighten your back. Breathe here.

The earth poses encourage a real physical sense of balance in the body. We often notice that one side of the body is tighter or weaker than the other. Yoga will eventually bring both sides back to equilibrium – if we persevere with our practice and be patient.

Water exercise – Cobra (bhujangasana) / Happy baby pose (ananda balasana)

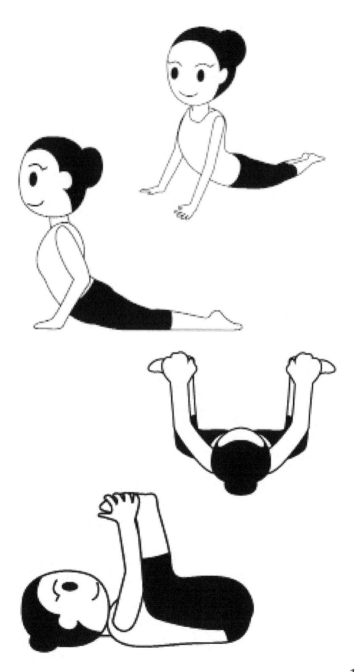

The cobra is a strengthening pose for the lower back, buttocks and shoulders and a really great stretch for the thighs, hips, stomach and throat.

- Begin the pose lying on your stomach. Bring your legs straight and together
- Bring your feet, and heels together.
- Make sure your hands are flat to the ground underneath the shoulders
- Tuck the elbows in and squeeze the shoulder blades together and downwards (towards the central spine)
- Engage the buttocks and stomach as you lift your chest off the floor. Look up and breathe through the belly three times before releasing back to the ground.

When we feel tired and creatively deprived, cobra empowers us.

Come onto your back from cobra and try out the happy baby pose.

- Bend the knees, bring the legs off the floor and have the soles of the feet facing the ceiling.
- Get comfortable with the spine nice and flat on the ground
- Grip onto the sides or arches of the feet or, hook your fingers around the big toes. Feel the groin and perineum stretching and the lower back sinking into the ground.

Any movement or flow encouraged in the hip region such as dancing, helps us release fears and experience joy again.

Fire exercise – Sitting head to knee forward bend (janu sirsasana) and spinal twist (ardha matsyendrasana)

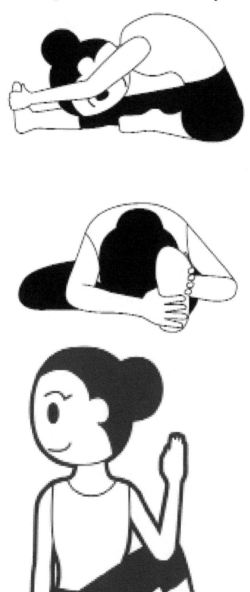

The forward bend and twist sequences are the ultimate internal massage for the small and large intestines, stomach, liver, spleen, pancreas, kidneys and bladder. These poses not only strengthen our core, they cleanse out the toxicity in the organs and stoke our fire energy to aid healthy peristalsis (digestion).

- Sit on the floor with one leg in front of you and the other leg bent at the knee, placing the sole of that foot against the opposite inner thigh.

- Engage with your core strength but also lift your heart to protect your back from overarching.
- Come into the forward bend slowly as you keep the stomach muscles engaged and relax the neck. Bring the arms along the legs and hold the calf muscle, ankle or toe. Stay in the pose for three deep breaths. Release, swap legs and repeat on the other side
- From the forward bend you can come into the twist by moving the bent leg upright and placing the sole of the foot on the floor.
- Take your opposite arm over the bent leg. Placing the back of the upper arm onto the outside of the knee/thigh. Place your free hand on the floor behind you for support – without leaning back.
- Engage in the spinal twist for three deep breaths. Release and repeat on the other side.

These poses are so effective for rebooting our energy. Note - you don't have to get your head to your leg, or twist around like an owl on the first go. Yoga is about the journey, not the destination!

Air exercise – bow (dhanurasana) / fish (matsyasana)

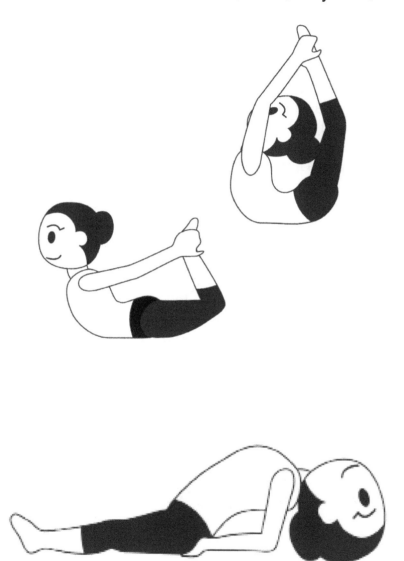

The bow bending and heart sequences are often experienced as the nemesis poses. I recommend being guided through these by a teacher.

In our modern lifestyle we often internally rotate our posture, through computer work, driving and sitting; going against what nature intended. Bow bends can feel awkward and uncomfortable and this is exactly why we need to practice them. Notice that children get into these poses intuitively.

Working on our flexibility in this area can encourage an openness and connection with our inner child as well as feeling all the neglected antagonistic muscles in action as they are engaged and contracted.

Launching into these poses too soon can cause injury. Bow bending and heart opening poses must be practiced slowly and with caution. When we master them, it is truly liberating.

Space exercise – shoulder stand (sarvangasana) and head stand (sirsasana)

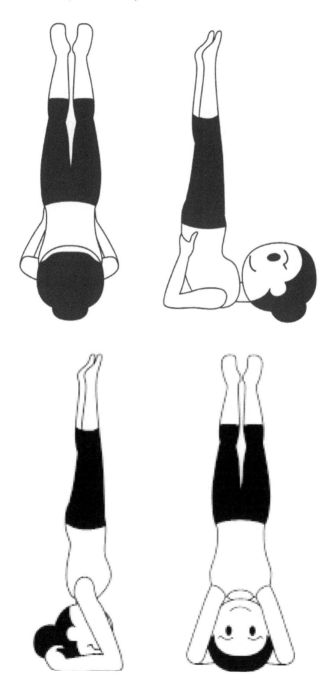

The shoulder and head stand poses are the king and queen of yoga poses. An internal massage for the heart, lungs, throat and brain. The ultimate in traditional hatha asana practice. When learned and practiced correctly our whole entity is encompassed with rushing energy and awakening. This can cause our egos to become very inflated though! When practiced incorrectly, there can be serious injury and a humble apology from your ego will be greatly appreciated by your 'self'. I recommend being guided through these by a teacher.

If these poses feel too intense, begin by lying on the floor with your buttocks as close to the wall as possible, and then slowly walk your legs up the wall. Lay in this position for a minute and enjoy some relaxation. This pose is fantastic for our circulation and prepares the body to move into shoulder stand when you are ready.

Breath (pranayama) exercise -

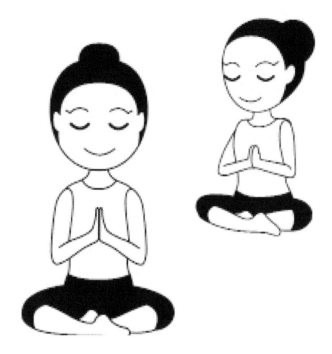

- With your fingers, place them gently on your beautiful face and begin to circle them around your eye orbits over and over again. Creating a wheel as you slowly breath in and out. Then raise your shoulders up and down at least five times as you breath in and out. Finally, place your left hand on your heart and your right hand on your burning belly and say to yourself...

'Breathe in self-love, breathe out self-doubt'.

It's time to get over yourself. To stop assuming. Stop trying to anticipate an outcome driven by fear of the unknown, because more than likely it won't be the one you are expecting. Stop expecting altogether. You are always one step ahead of yourself.

You do this for protection. To get ahead. To try and predict what is going to happen so that you can be ready, on defence, or ready to run. You may be experiencing a moment of catastrophe in your head brain and subsequently ignoring your heart and gut brains. You are experiencing human suffering because of immense over thinking and intellectualising.

Again – simply breathe in self-love, breathe out self-doubt...Your breath is your guide. Your internal navigation system to your power, truth and the stillness within.

Step 4 – Fuel

You are feeding the source

Ayurveda meaning 'knowledge of life' is a well-respected Indian science which predominantly focuses on preventative medicine practice. Rather than our more familiar modern medical system designed to treat and cure symptoms.

According to the Bhagavad Gita, (a section of verses from one of the major Sanskrit scriptures) the yogic diet is summarized into three main qualities.

PURE - Sattvic foods – *'The foods which increase life, purity, strength, health, joy and cheerfulness, which are savoury and oleaginous, substantial and agreeable, are dear to the sattvic people.'* **Bhagavad Gita, XVII,8**

OVER - STIMULATING - Rajasic foods – *'Foods that are bitter, sour, saline, excessively hot, pungent, dry and burning, are liked by the rajasic and are productive of pain, grief and disease.'* **Bhagavad Gita, XVII,9**

PUTREFIED - Tamasic foods – *'That food which is stale, tasteless, putrid, rotten and impure refuse, is the food liked by the tamasic.'* **Bhagavad Gita, XVII,10**

Sattvic foods make up a lacto-vegetarian diet that not only fuels our physical machine with essential nutrients, but also contains the subtlest energy which aids and supports the construct of our mind. Sattvic food frees the body from dis-ease and dis-order so that the mind can focus, and the spirit can develop. Continued practice of the many arms of yoga will eventually encourage you to choose sattvic food. It is suggested that continuing to

161

choose rajasic and tamasic food will hinder your mental make-up, toxicity and eventually cause disease.

If we look deeper, Ayurveda & Yogic science talks of preserving and maximising our natural dosha (body type). Ultimately sattvic food suitable to the natural dosha is the key to doing this. If, however the dosha is aggravated or depleted in any way it might be necessary to encourage re-balance with a wider range of prescribed herbs and foods in order to achieve dosha balance again. A dosha analysis is a great tool in helping us make the best choices for our holistic health, starting with the food we eat.

We are born with a dominant dosha and over time our exposure to various environmental, social and emotional changes disturb our natural body constitution. When our dominant dosha and our chakra system are re-balanced we have a great chance at discovering 'WHOLE' health and wellness and preventing inflammation and disease.

Exercise –

Below is a list of each dosha and their qualities/ imbalances along with the foods suited to the body type. Consult our expert at iamwellnesssolution@ gmail.com if you would like a detailed ayurvedic analysis.

Which dosha do you resonate with?

....
A dosha taster…

VATA = The creator
PITTA = The action taker
KAPHA = The preserver

Vata dosha qualities –
- Naturally creative
- Light physique
- Dry skin

Signs of aggravation in vata –
- Worry
- Constipation
- Dehydration

Optimal food choice for vata –
- Root teas such as ginger and liquorice
- Mild spices
- Ripe fruits and starchy vegetables

Pitta dosha qualities –
- Productive
- Medium physique
- Fair skin

Signs of aggravation in pitta –
- Irritation
- Diarrhoea
- Excess sweating

Optimal food choice for pitta –
- Cooling teas such as peppermint and chamomile
- Cooling spices such as cumin, mint, coriander
- Sweet fruit and raw or steamed vegetables

Kapha dosha qualities –
- Logical
- Substantial physique
- Oily skin

Signs of aggravation in kapha –
- Procrastination
- Sluggish bowels
- Fungal and bacterial infections

Optimal food choice for kapha -
- Strong spices such as pepper, mustard, tumeric
- Cleansing teas such as raspberry and green
- Ripe citrus fruits, steamed vegetables and non-starchy grains

We are seeing the benefits that Ayurveda and Yoga have on our ever-increasing modern-day stresses. Yoga practice, traditional massage, and dosha nutrition tailored to the individual goes a long way in preventing and alleviating many health conditions. Consciously making the connection that sattvic food has a high vibrational quality, which in turn affects the health of our bio-energy field and our physical body is paramount in achieving optimum HOLISTIC well-being.

Step 5 – Self care

You are nourishing the head, heart and gut through the skin

The skin, also known as the integumentary system, is the largest organ in the body. It is the first line of defence against pathogenic attack to our internal organs. Some of the nerve pathways in the skin are connected directly to muscles instead of the brain so that we can respond more quickly to sensory exposure such as heat and pain. Plus the skin regulates our body temperature. Skin renews itself every 28-30 days and we shed approximately 40,000 dead skin cells per minute. We have roughly 20 square feet of skin which contains over 10 miles of blood vessels, 19 million cells and 300 sweat glands. Aside from all of this, the skin is the bridge between our physical mass and energetic vibration. When we love our skin, our heart is full and our entity is in balance.

Earth – salt

Using salt as a topical application is one of the most ancient and effective ways to exfoliate and detoxify the system, stimulating blood flow, removing dead skin cells and grounding mental activity. Himalayan, magnesium, epsom or sea salt blended with a simple vegetable oil such as olive, grapeseed or sesame oil will aid in shedding dead skin cells and bringing a natural glow back to our energy field.

Home remedy – 20 – 50 g chosen salt, 20 – 30 g chosen plant-based oil (avoid a pre-blend) and 3 drops of chosen citrus based essential oil (such as mandarin, orange or lemon oil*)

- Standing in the bath or shower on a non-slip mat, blend the ingredients into a small bowl with a non-metallic spoon.
- Apply the scrub in circular movements generously over the whole body for approximately 5-10 minutes before bathing or showering.
- Alternatively, sitting down with your feet on a towel, apply the scrub over the feet, toes, heels and lower leg for a pick-me up exfoliation.
- Rinse feet with warm water and pat dry with a towel.

Natural clay and seaweeds are other ingredients that are useful to ground our energy and revive tired skin. Clay skin care methods have been used for hundreds of years and work by drawing impurities out of the skin whilst soothing inflammation and regulating oil production. The most accessible clays and seaweeds for home remedy use are bentonite clay and chlorella algae.

Water – oil

The nourishing nature of pure lipid (fatty) oils not only feeds the skin with crucial hydration and moisture, but also encourage restrictive areas of soft tissue to loosen. Applying liberal amounts of oil to the face and body provided a healthy flow for lymphatic fluid and blood which supports the immune, cardio-vascular system and effectively eliminates waste product from the body.

Home remedy – Apply once a day or more if you have dry skin.

- Jojoba for the face
- Coconut for the hair
- Sweet almond, sesame and olive oil for the body

Fire – heat

Our solar plexus is a system of conversion. The activities of metabolising and digesting can be demanding. Bringing warmth to the stomach and middle back gently restores and regulates this area if it is under-active or over stimulated.

Home remedy - Hot water bottle or topical application once a week followed by a flame gazing meditation.

A topical application of a heating balm such as tiger or ayurvedic pain balm helps to regulate the solar plexus. The general rule with balm products is 'a little goes a long way'.

- Rubbing a small amount into the upper stomach in a spiral motion and then applying into the middle back is the ideal remedy for releasing stomach gases or reviving a depleted digestive system.

Ingesting peppermint and liqourice teas regularly, will support the healthy functioning of the gastro-intestinal system.

Trataka is a Sanskrit word for 'gaze'. This form of meditation is done with the eyes open unlike traditional meditation.

- Use a small object or flame and gaze at it for 5 – 10 minutes a day, our eyes and mind learn to focus and our vital energy is restored.

As sight is the corresponding sense for the fire/solar plexus centre, exercising our gaze is a healthy practice and is also said to open our third eye awareness.

Air – steam

Steaming the full body or the head under a towel is the most active way to open up the lungs, relieve tightness in the chest and remove stale air from deep within the bronchiole (tubes) and alveoli (air sacks). Steaming is a great defense against illness and doesn't have to be saved until we get sick. Consciously steaming once a week with therapeutic essential oils offers preventative cleansing and is also a great way to relieve grief and stress, supporting the healing of your heart.

My top three essential oils for steaming-

- *Rosemary -stimulant, sudorific (increases perspiration to aid cleansing)

- *Eucalyptus – anti-inflammatory, antispasmodic (preventing cramps and spasms)

- *Lavender – decongestant, antidepressant (relieves and reduces mucous)

Home remedy– 4 drops of rosemary, 4 drops of lavender and 3 drops of eucalyptus

For a steam bowl –

- Find a stable surface and fill a large bowl with 2 parts boiling water and 1 part cold water.
- Add the essential oil blend into the water.
- Sit comfortably, place a towel over your head and lean over the bowl. Carefully enclose the towel leaving a small gap for excess steam to release.
- Steam for up to 15 minutes with intervals every 4-5 minutes.

For shower or bath-

- Wet a cloth with warm water and drop the oils directly on top of each other so they soak into the surface.
- Place the cloth on the side of the bath and start running the bath so that the steam releases the therapeutic scent.
- Once the bath has been drawn, immerse the cloth into the water. (Do not rub cloth directly onto your skin as this may cause irritation).

Space – sound and ingest

Experiencing sound wave healing will directly home in on the sense of hearing associated with the ether centre at a deep vibrational level. The high quality of sound healing not only calms mental activity but supports thyroid function and overall cellular rejuvenation. Flooding the auditory system with Sanskrit mantra's and chanting provides a different kind of music to the ears. One that is designed to unlock spiritual potential and expression.

This would be an optimal time to document your reflections in a gratitude journal. Writing one page every day is a healthy way to express yourself. If you are not ready to communicate through sound and voice, start with ink and paper.

- To complete the final stage of the five rituals I recommend drinking a herbal tonic which supports gut health and inevitably skin health. Plants such as **ashwagandha, **turmeric and **neem are traditional to the Indian health sciences and are vital herbs in integumentary support.

*Do not use essential oils on cuts, rashes, broken skin or directly after shaving as this may cause irritation. Do not ingest essential oils. Avoid contact with eyes and mucous membranes. Seek professional medical advice if volatile oils make contact with eyes, mucous membranes or are ingested.

**Do not ingest herbal tonics without instructions from a professional therapist or practitioner. Do not use if you are pregnant, trying to conceive, having I.V.F, breastfeeding, have diabetes or un-medicated high blood pressure.

YOU ARE UNRAVELLING

'Don't build a wall around your own suffering – it may devour you from the inside'

Frida Kahlo

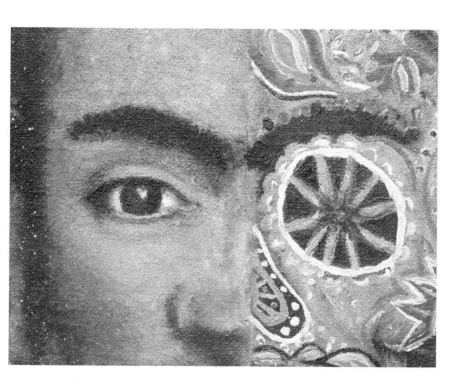

Exploring some of the poignant examples in my life where I have experienced trauma or a major change in circumstances that felt out of my control, is often where I have discovered a sense of liberation through life experiences, self-development and spiritual practice. As a child, as a traveller, giving birth, during my yoga and transformation training and with my clients – who have taught me so much.

One thing that remains consistent throughout, is that life will continue to throw something else on the path whether it be good or bad. So, whenever my anxiety and fear creep up on me, I actively look to reconnect with that openness and space within my own internal universe. Seeking the truth. Learning, rather than deflecting or rejecting growth. When I do, all the made-up stress produced in my mind and body, begins to shed off me again. Then, more stuff comes along and I remind myself to stop, reconnect with my internal universe and then shed another layer and another. Always exposing the truth. It is a process, a journey, not a one-stop fix-it shop.

Peeling back these layers feels revealing and uncomfortable. We often associate the word unravelling with 'falling apart' but it can be a very productive word too. Being absolutely truthful with yourself and others takes courage, which might be why we don't often go there! If we have many lies to come face-to-face with and rectify, this process may take some time but it is a step in the direction of cleaning up our karma. By releasing the fear we have around people and circumstances, we no longer have to hide and live in the shadows of ourselves. Shedding the old to explore what spaces open up can be daunting and time consuming. We have to begin to make small shifts in our daily life to make a 'truth' practice attainable. When we do this, we learn to be humble and gracious.

Reminding ourselves that energy is in a constant state of flux, always changing and forming in new ways based on how we act, think and feel about every single part of our lives, we can really understand the power of our own energy force within our physical container. If we grasp the idea of cause and effect and take responsibility of every untruth that we hold about ourselves and every little lie we have presented to others, we begin to generate that powerful force. Combining our internal force with our full self-expression is the elixir of honesty that we can now offer to the world; the beginning of living with integrity and causing a beautiful and healing ripple effect.

Are you at the effect or the cause of your life?

Do you feel empowered to add your elixir to the wild, flowing river and JUMP IN! Or, are you helpless and getting swept up in the current?

Let's get into a space where we put all of that 'stuff' 'talk' 'habits' to one side for a moment. A space where the physical body and the mind are unified. When we start to gauge that our body and mind are working as one, we can begin to explore the other dimension to our being, the space of healing, peace and real human potential.

When I assist my physical body with self-care and healing rituals I come back into alignment with my peaceful clearing. My 'knowing'. One works in hand with the other and to identify with your own calm and peace in life you must do some internal work and self-examination. We must experience a moment for ourselves where we know truth (without necessarily knowing or being told), where expectations, fabrications, fight, resistance and a need to follow our sensory desires, is no longer a priority or default for us.

Exploring what your true reset button looks like is the first step to a commitment to your self-care. My go to reset button are my rituals. My daily reminders to come back to living with my truth. Other activities I commit to are regular thai massage therapy, regular time spent being in stillness (even if I have to block it out in the diary) and equally movement. I love to dance for example, especially with children. They are a beautiful example of truthful expression in action. We all have our own variations of this because we have learned what to do to stay healthy and well over and over again: Exercising, eating well, good sleep and good company.

Yet, most of us don't seem to stick to this consistently. Why? Maybe we find ourselves bumbling through: Following trends, keen to keep up the pursuit of looking good at the cost of our integrity. Some of us will do this for the rest of our days until we die. This may be within the realms of 'just fine'. And if that is the case then those people are probably not interested in reading this. For others, this does not sit well. For others this might not feel like 'what it's all about'. Maybe you are one of the ones who are curious; the ones that go looking for that crack of light; someone who wants to inquire more deeply into their life.

First and foremost, we have to honour what our truth is. As you read this is it making you feel excited to explore your truth or uncomfortable? Ask yourself that question now and document it. Why do you feel excited or uncomfortable?

....

....

....

....

If you are unsure what is coming up for you it is sometimes useful to look at this in a different scenario. For example, whether we are being truthful with ourselves in the physical world.

Do you go to that gym class because you really want to or because you feel you have too? Start to explore the healthy things you enjoy doing instead of being herded along to that circuit class that you hate! (Note – you may love a circuit class. I do not love a circuit class.)

When you discover what you genuinely enjoy you can choose for this to be your reset button. When you know what your reset button is, own it, share it and do it with integrity and freedom of expression.

Your truth will be very different from one person to the next, so we must honour that but certainly not compromise ourselves so much that it becomes detrimental to our balance.   In fact, when we become honestly aligned with ourselves we are much more willing to accept other's reset buttons with the utmost respect rather than thinking they are wrong for doing their 'thing'.

Once you get into the habit of that fun, healthy reset button that you genuinely love doing this will propel you onto a path of the highest vibrational energy. This is the optimum environment for acceptance of others, confidence in speaking truthfully regardless of the fear you feel, and your openness to explore your internal universe.

YOU ARE A UNIVERSE

'Nothing is impossible, the word itself says I'm-possible'

Audrey Hepburn.

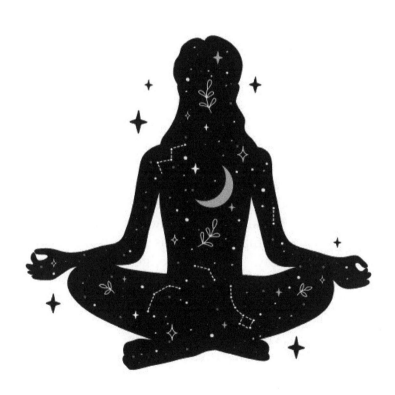

Spending a lot of time in nature is a great way for me to connect to my clear space in times of upheaval. During my travels is where this was extremely heightened. Standing at the foot of a mountain range or the edge of a glacier I became acutely aware of how small my physical body was in this vast universal space made up of earth, water, fire and air. This is all there really is: The five elements showing up in different forms in our cosmos.

As I explored the knowledge of the elements, I began to see the direct connection between our physical body and all things naturally occurring on earth and in our cosmos. As I zoom out my personal perspective lens even further, I can see that what we humans know about our solar system and the universe also correlates directly with the functions and rhythms of our physical body.

Our micro matter (the stuff that makes up our physical world, as a matter of scientific fact) is identical to the same matter that makes up our universe. Both the ancient yogis and modern -day scientists are in agreement with this. When I really got this concept and the penny dropped, I remember feeling as though mankind just had an epiphany. This knowledge is truly incredible and needs to be shared and why wasn't anyone talking about it? Why didn't I learn this in school?

Having always been tactile and inclined kinaesthetically it's no wonder I wanted to explore the study of integrated body therapy. I spent a lot of time learning anatomy and physiology and alongside this, the science of our bio energy field.

The cellular structure of a plant is made up of the same stuff as our body's cells. The healing qualities in plants, whether it be from the root, the stem, the flower or the fruit, can enhance the recovery time of our cells and give our bodies the nutrients and components it needs to function optimally and bring back ultimate balance for an array of physical and mental conditions. All holistic healing modalities (from lymphatic drainage, craniosacral therapy, myofascial release, chakra balancing, Ayurveda, TCM) fundamentally support our body's ability to heal and flow. Isn't this what we are designed to do: move and flow?

The idea that there is more to us than the physical body is second nature to me now. I firmly believe that our human body wasn't designed to go to work at a desk nearly every day for 50 years. It is far from intelligent to spend an average 90,000 hours of our life at work. There are more important and powerful things to discover.

Our busy 21st century lifestyle doesn't align with our simple purpose of obtaining an awakening of peace and love in our life and solidarity with others. Our ultimate goal is not to achieve material success with accolades and certificates that re-enforce how we identify with ourselves and our success, but rather to obtain a oneness with ourselves, a spiritual fulfilment and a unity with our fellow human and natural world on a deep, authentic, connected level.

I have aided so much of my own healing or been the receiver of remarkable shifts in my physical pain and emotional suffering as well as facilitating many people in theirs too. We are essentially made of the five universal elements, five senses, intellect and underneath all that-huge potential. To thrive as humans, we simply need to nurture these elements within us, have them in balance, and move through our life with a firm sense of being. Immovable from our truth yet flexible and flowing enough to remain open and unaffected by external influence and pressure. The saying ' We are all made of stars' is not to be laughed at because we truly are. When we accept and connect with this simple concept of the five elements and our chakra energy system, we really do have the power to self-care, self-love and preserve our physical and emotional selves from unnecessary drama and suffering in many areas of our life. Family, relationships, work, kids, friends, social life, social structure.

The external system we live in, the way we form our identity and beliefs and understanding of the world is all essentially made up from our intellectual, social and economic perspective. This is not saying that we should reject the material world we live in, rather learn to be unattached to any sense of being trapped in it. When you become open to peeling back your identity within an existing social construct there will be an opening in you, where no limits exist. If we think about the existing social framework in which we live, we know that we humans created it. In order to create something; we must have had the idea in the first place and then believed in it enough to get others on board, create a sense of community to help us expand our ideas into fruition. Isn't that incredible in itself? That humans have achieved such great creations in time, all because they captured a feeling of what was possible and ran with it? So, if that happened back then, what can we humans do now?

Humans are our best selves when we have a greater sense of self without labels and expectations, when we have heightened compassion for others and a drive to stand in our truth and express it in all areas of our life.

Now, give yourself permission to be you. Standing inside of your potential and not chained or governed by your own limitations or any of the limitations that you may feel have been set on you. Do the thing and be the person you always wanted to be and then watch what manifests. You don't deserve to be resigned in your life. You can design your life, all you need is an idea, a brush and a blank canvas -this is your clearing, right in front of you.

'YOU ARE '

*'The meaning of life is to find
your gift. The purpose of life
is to give it away.'*

Pablo Picasso.

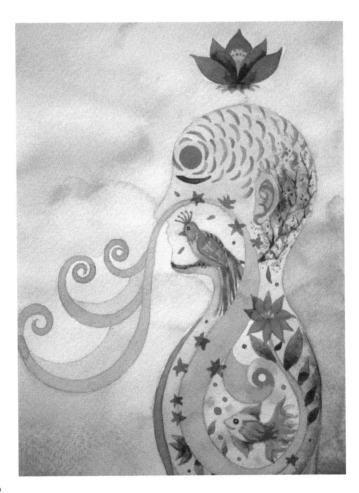

What are you going to give out today?

Noise - Space and sound - when I am 'on one' and my mouth won't shut up gossiping and judging others.

Hostility - Air and touch – when I am being stingy with my affection and not allowing myself to receive love.

Abuse - Fire and sight – when I am consuming unhealthy food and drink as a way of punishing myself for the unworthiness I see.

Consumption - Water and taste – when I am not moving enough, restricted and limited by fear and desire.

Indecision - Earth and smell – when I am not able to be still and trusting of the ground I walk on.

When I am being this way, I have low energy, low thoughts, low mood and minimal contribution to my loved ones, my community and humankind. I am being stagnant, rotten and useless in this space. Plodding through life, entitled, egocentric and driven only by empty desires. Ultimately suffering.

Who shall we be today?

A listening ear - Space and sound – when I get up out of bed, actively affirm GREAT language and gratitude for my life and listen openly and calmly to others.

Compassionate - Air and touch – when I hug, love, compliment others and share myself.

Respectful - Fire and sight – when I sustainably receive mother earth's plants and berries for energy and goodness.

Free - Water and taste – when I get moving through joy not duty and let go of my addictive tendencies.

Grateful - Earth and smell – when I get out into nature with my feet firmly on the ground making a stand for my life.

When I am being this way, I experience a clearing in front of me. I am now brave enough to step into it. I know no physical limitations here. In this space I am free and fulfilled with a deep sense that anything is possible for myself, my life and my fellow human, whoever you are, wherever you are, whatever you have and do - you and I are universally connected....

Hello human

I AM willing and **I AM** worthy of
my greatness today!

Who are you?

Begin your **I AM** journey, discover your
inner therapist and realise your greatness!

References

- Sivananda yoga teachers training manual
- Man's Greatest Adventure – Paramahansa Yogananda, Self Realization International Head Quarters, Los Angeles, California-February 29th 1940. Published in 'Man's Eternal Quest'.
- The Complete Guide to Aromatherapy – Salvatore Battaglia
- Ayurveda for Spa and Wellness, A comprehensive introductory program by Tri-Dosha Ayurvedic training academy
- The Landmark Forum Curriculum
- Simply psychology.com
- You Can Heal Your Life – Louise L Hay
- The Power of Now, A guide to spiritual enlightenment - Eckhart Tolle
- Global Wellness Institute research centre
- Chris Day - Filament Publishing Ltd
- Biography.com
- Principles of Anatomy and Physiology by Gerald J. Tortora and Bryan Derrickson. 11th Edition

Join the member's area-
access your free audio meditation
or enrol on the
I AM WELLness 25-day plan here -
carlychamberlain.podia.com

Join the community- @carlyiamwellness
Work with me - iamwellnesssolution@gmail.com /
linkedin.com/in/carly-chamberlain /
Facebook - @carlychamberlainwellness